made
millie mackintosh

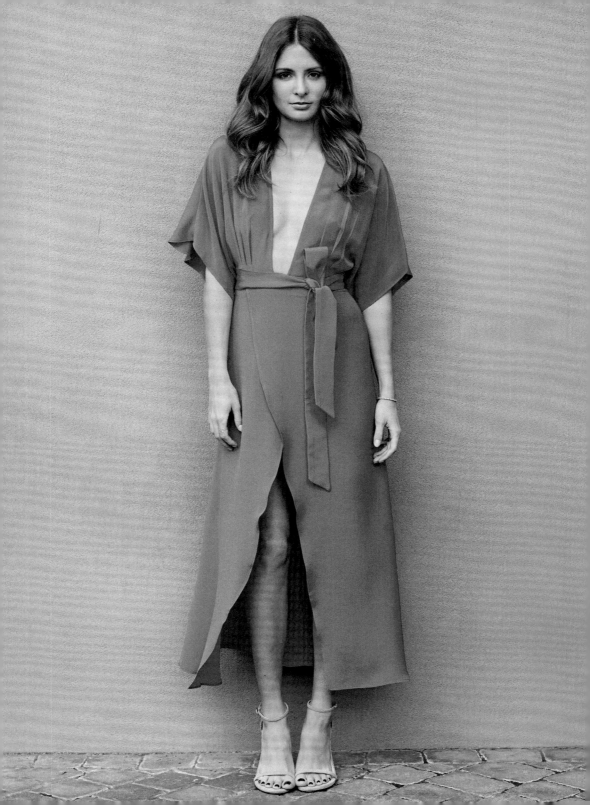

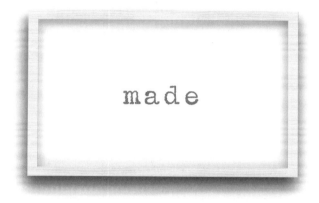

made

millie mackintosh

EBURY
PRESS

FOR JENNIFER WARD 1937–2002, MY MATERNAL GRANNY,
AND FELICITY MACKINTOSH 1931–, MY PATERNAL GRANNY,
FOR ALWAYS SUPPORTING AND INSPIRING ME X

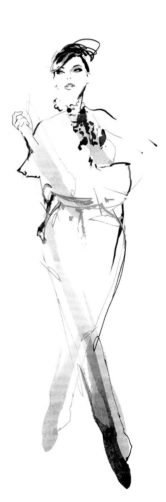

1 0 9 8 7 6 5 4 3 2

Ebury Press, an imprint of Ebury Publishing,
20 Vauxhall Bridge Road, London, SW1V 2SA

Ebury Press is part of the Penguin Random House group of companies
whose addresses can be found at global.penguinrandomhouse.com

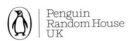

Penguin
Random House
UK

First published by Ebury Press in 2015

www.eburypublishing.co.uk

A CIP catalogue record for this book is available from the British Library

Design: Smith & Gilmour
Photography: Daniel Kennedy
Illustrations: Francesca Waddell
Food and prop stylist: Emma Lahaye

ISBN: 9781785030819

Colour origination by Altaimage, London.
Printed and bound by Firmengruppe APPL, aprinta druck, Wemding, Germany.

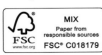

contents

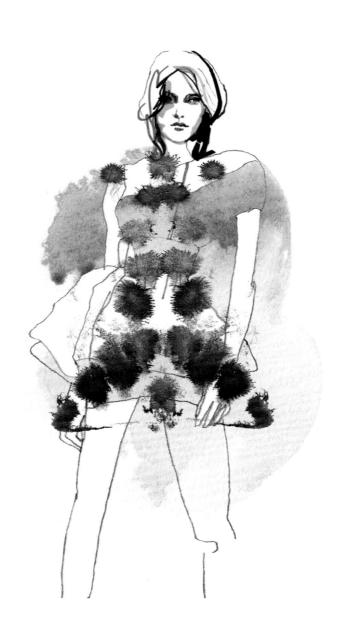

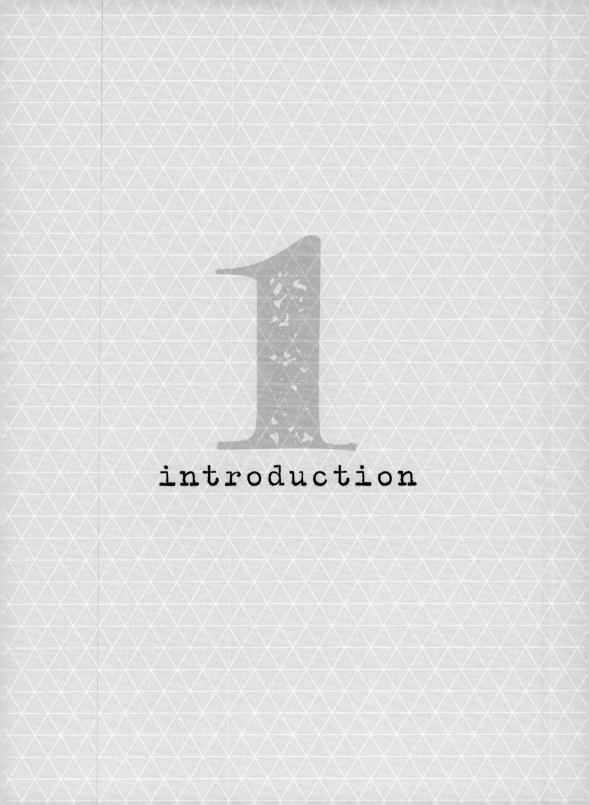

1

introduction

Sunday 27 May 2012 was the moment I realised that my life had changed. I was standing on a Union Jack carpet in a white Lanvin dress at the television BAFTAs with Stephen, the *Made in Chelsea* cast and a whole load of other people I had only ever seen on the TV. As the cameras flashed, I remember thinking how surreal it all was: a year ago, no one had heard of me.

Being famous had never been on my to-do list. As a child, I'd had phases of wanting to be a Disney princess, a ballerina, a vet and a model, but a reality TV star? I didn't even know what that was!

My arrival in the world could hardly be described as glamorous. I was born in Swindon hospital on a Wednesday afternoon in July 1989 – the 26th, to be precise – and my parents named me Camilla Margaret. No one has called me Camilla since; I've always been Milla to my family and I reinvented myself as Millie when I arrived at secondary school at the age of 12. I thought it sounded more sophisticated. Mum remembers a teacher talking to her about a girl called Millie and not realising she was talking about me!

I wanted to consolidate all the things I've learned and to pass them on. I'm not saying that this is the only way, or even the best way; it's just what works for me

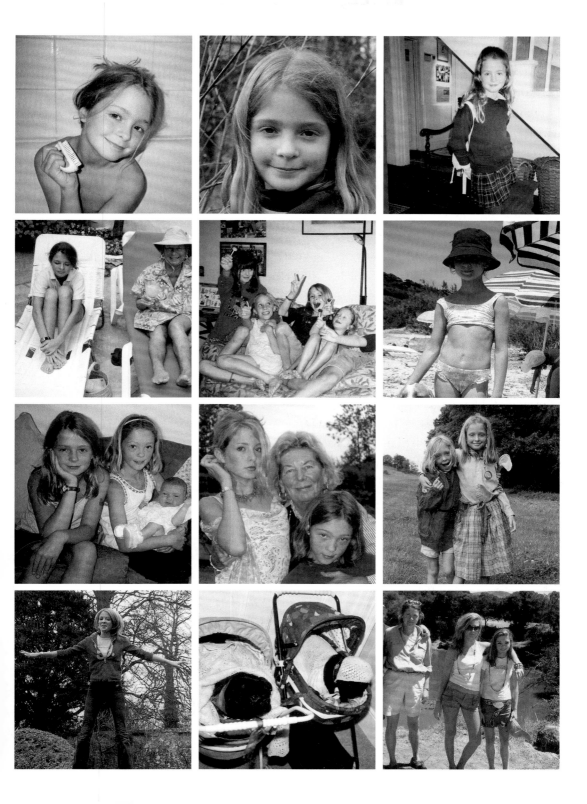

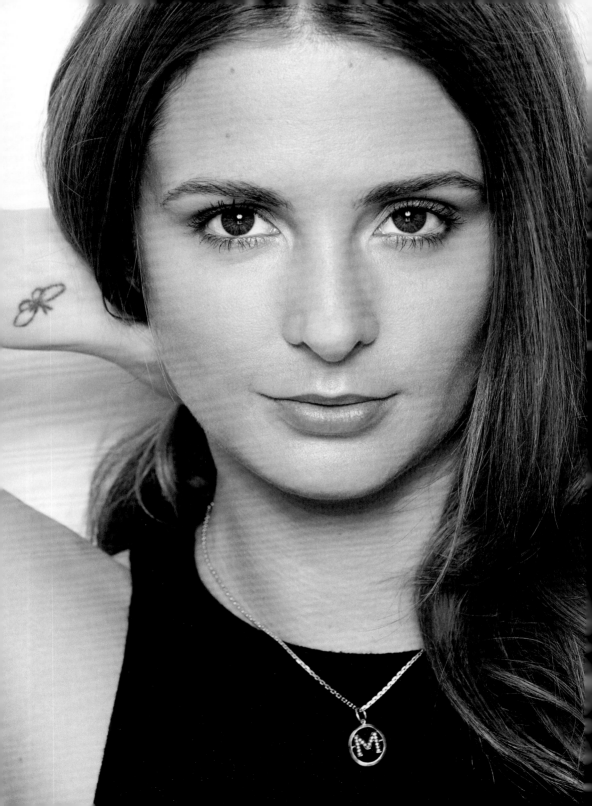

Home was an old vicarage in a tiny Wiltshire village called Milton Lilbourne and our garden had a meadow and lots of trees to climb. It was idyllic – all tree houses and paddling pools – and I spent lots of time playing outside. Most weekends were spent going on long country walks and there were always picnics in the summer.

Following fashion wasn't my thing as a child – it wasn't even on my radar – but I did love fancy dress. My sister Alice was crazy about the rocking horse we had, but for me the best thing in the house was the dressing-up box. There was a tutu that I'd wear underneath another skirt to make it puff out, a Princess Jasmine costume from *Aladdin* and a 1980s Versace chain-print dress of my mum's which I adored.

I was mad about make-up too. I loved watching my mum and my two very glamorous grannies getting ready to go out. Fascinated by the transformative power of all the products on their dressing tables, I soon had a stash of my own; I remember being particularly proud of a trio of eye shadows and some telephone-box red Chanel nail varnish.

At eight, I was sent to an all-girls boarding school in Dorset. It was a bit like *St Trinian's*; we weren't quite as badly behaved as that, though there were booby traps in the dormitories and midnight feasts. And we spent a lot of time riding ponies. Fashion wasn't even on our radar. However, I had no idea quite how uncool I was until I started secondary school. It was another boarding school for girls, but of a rather more worldly kind: the first person I saw when I arrived was a pupil in skin-tight Miss Sixty hipster jeans, a belly-button piercing and a boob tube cropped short enough to show it off. My mum was horrified, but I thought she looked fantastic. Standing there in my baggy Gap fleece, I decided that I wanted to be just like her.

It wasn't easy for me. I was lanky, awkward and flat-chested, with a brace, bad skin, glasses and frizzy hair. I remember one of the older girls giving me a makeover before the year nine school social. (These

were a big deal because they involved boys from a nearby school.)
She lent me her mini kilt, a pair of heels (my first) and did my hair
with straighteners she'd borrowed from one of the other girls. (Hair
straighteners were new then and only a few kids had them; they
rented them out at £5 a go.) For the first few hours, the girls stayed
on one side of the hall and the boys on the other, but when the last,
slow, song came on, everyone immediately found someone to dance
with. Including me. I had my first kiss to Robbie Williams's 'Angels'.
I remember it tasted of Sprite!

My school days weren't a very happy time for me. I'm dyspraxic,
which means I have spatial-awareness problems, so I was never
picked for any of the sports teams. I was quite badly bullied too;
people teased me because I was skinny with big feet. (I'm a size six,
but my feet are flat and long and sensible school shoes just looked
like boats on me; my parents wouldn't let me have the cool ones with
a heel. These days I hardly ever wear flats.) But eventually I found
a bunch of friends I could be myself around and life at school got
much better. I remember one of my friends telling me that the

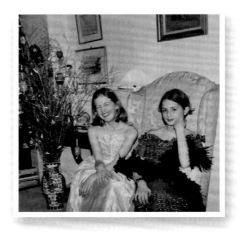

reason a particular group of girls always picked on me was because they were really insecure themselves and teasing me made them feel powerful. That totally changed the way I thought about them and helped me to see that it was the bullies who had the problems, not me. Knowing that helped me to ignore them.

By the age of 16, my social life was in London. I was doing a BTEC diploma in Art and Design at a mixed boarding school in Somerset, but lots of my friends from my previous schools had homes in London and I would go up at any opportunity, escaping at the weekend as often as I could. My girlfriends and I would hang out in Chelsea and go off clubbing dressed in the most indecent clothes ever – tiny mini dresses and heels we couldn't walk in. I remember various parents suggesting that we wore coats, but we thought we were far too cool for that. It makes my face burn now to think about some of those outfits!

I've always really loved the buzz and excitement of London – you can feel it as soon as you get off the train – so when I left school, that was where I headed. I had this idea that I wanted to be a make-up

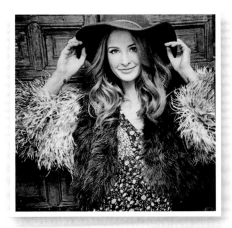

artist – I'd had a temp job with MAC one Christmas, which I really enjoyed – so when I got back from my post-sixth form travels, I did an eight-week course and, after lots of rejections, finally got a job at Space NK. It was great experience; I had to do make-up on all sorts of different faces every day and I learned a lot about skin care in the process. I wasn't that bothered about making sales, but what I did enjoy was helping people solve their skin-care or make-up problems. I remember one girl came in with very troublesome skin and I recommended a few products and a cleansing routine and two weeks later she came back to show me how much better she looked. I was so pleased. It was fun doing makeovers too, but some of the customers were incredibly rude. I got foundation on this woman's white coat by accident once; she went crazy.

The job was fine but as I didn't like working on the shop floor, I knew retail wasn't for me and I wasn't absolutely sure that I wanted to be a make-up artist either. I was quite interested in modelling and I'd auditioned for the television show *Britain's Next Top Model* (I failed the 'best catwalk walk' test in front of Elle 'The Body' Macpherson and Julien MacDonald, so didn't make it to the live rounds), but like many 20-year-olds, I didn't have a very clear sense of where I was heading career-wise. And then along came *Made in Chelsea*.

It happened by chance really. I was living with one of my best friends near the New King's Road and one evening I was at home getting ready for a date. I yelled across the corridor to ask whether my flatmate thought thigh-high boots were a bit much for a first date, and when she didn't answer, I hurtled into the sitting room with a long boot on one leg and an ankle boot on the other (not a great look), only to be greeted by two strange women who turned out to be the producers of the TV series, come to see my flatmate. I stayed long enough to get my answer (thigh-high boots) and left. For some reason, that rather embarrassing meeting appealed to the producers and a few days later they called to ask me if I was interested in appearing on the show.

At that stage, I wasn't at all sure that I wanted to take part. The idea definitely appealed to my exhibitionist side, but I was also anxious about getting roped into something that I would later regret. And what if everyone hated me? Then my flatmate decided she didn't want to be involved after all and the programme makers asked me if I had any other friends who they could meet. I immediately thought of Caggie Dunlop. Best friends since we were 16, we went travelling across Australia, Bali and Thailand after we left school and got into all kinds of scrapes. There was the time when Caggie got bitten by a rabid dog while she was jogging along the beach in Thailand. Rushing her to this pretty basic hospital facility was pretty scary. And then there was the skinny-dipping episode on Fraser Island, off the coast of Queensland, Australia. We were camping there and had been told not to swim but we decided to go anyway. A man appeared and started shouting at us but we ignored him, thinking he was just some creep who'd seen our discarded bikinis. However, when we got out we soon discovered our mistake – he'd been trying to tell us that it was the sharks' mating season! Back home we made a pact that we should always have our adventures together, so since neither of us really had a career at the time, we decided that we'd give *Made in Chelsea* a go. After all, what did we have to lose?

The first few programmes, which aired during the summer of 2011, were like a dream. We'd been filming for ages, but I still couldn't imagine it being on the television until it actually was. The whole cast gathered at the Soho Hotel to see the first episode. Watching myself on screen was horrendous (it still is), but by the time the third one aired, the show was getting lots of press, people were stopping me in the street and I was being asked to do interviews and shoots.

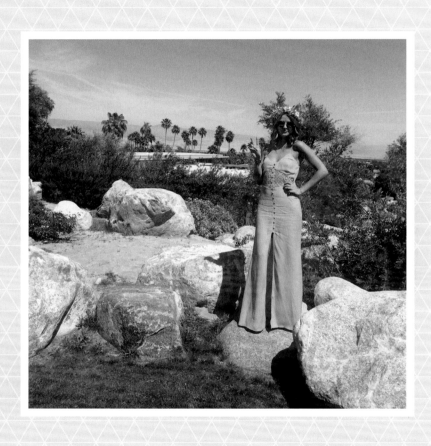

Looking back, I am grateful that I did it. Being on the show boosted my confidence and that enabled me to have a go at so many of the things I'd always wanted to do, like launching a range of false eyelashes, modelling and setting up my own clothing line. And I did have lots of fun times. I had a reputation for being quite feisty (if you watched the show, you'll know what I mean!), but one of the worst moments was when they filmed Caggie coming into *Glamour* magazine with a bottle of champagne. I was interning there and had no idea that the whole thing was a set-up for the show, so when the editor shouted at me for inviting my friends to the office, I thought I was going to be fired. That was a hairy moment, I can tell you, but then everyone started laughing and I realised I'd been set up.

But there were stressful times too – breaking up with someone on camera was particularly horrible – and I started to suffer from disabling anxiety attacks. I'd get palpitations, waves of nausea and this all-consuming sense of fear. I remember having one while we were filming at Nikki Beach in Marrakesh and then one of the producers told me to look at my feet and tell her where they were. I said they were standing in the sand and she replied, 'Well, if they're both on the ground then you're fine, aren't you?' I found that really helpful. I still get anxiety attacks from time to time and asking myself that question is a strategy that I continue to use to calm myself down.

I'd always promised myself that I would leave *Made in Chelsea* when I stopped enjoying it, or when it stopped being a success (it's always better to leave on a high). It wasn't such fun once Caggie left, and then I met Stephen. I knew I didn't want to have another relationship on screen, so I'd been planning to tell the producers I was leaving, but Stephen got there first. He announced it during an interview on Radio 1!

Life has been a whirlwind since then. I had already launched my false-eyelash range with Nouveau Lashes, but afterwards I got to do lots of modelling, appeared on *Celebrity MasterChef* (I love cooking but doing it under those conditions was terrifying) and then, in 2014, I set up a fashion line under my own name.

I had been asked to collaborate with a few fashion brands before, but I really wanted to do my own thing and create a clothing collection that reflected my trademark style. I have been completely hands-on at every stage because this isn't just something I'm putting my face to; it's my own brand. I began by creating lots of mood boards, bringing in some favourite pieces from my own wardrobe as inspiration, and then, because I've never been to fashion school, I worked with a team of experts to collate the designs, choose fabrics and come up with first samples. It's been quite tough – I've had to learn everything from how fabric falls to how to run a business – but I've enjoyed it and I am proud of the collections. I set out to create some must-have pieces and I think that's what I've achieved.

Meeting Stephen has made a big difference to my life, of course. It doesn't sound very romantic – and it absolutely wasn't set up or

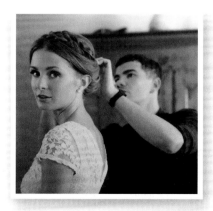

planned – but he got my phone number from his publicist. I'd done a cover photo for *FHM* and a copy of the magazine was lying around at a shoot he was on. He joked that he'd like to meet me, and his publicist she said that she could get my number from a mutual acquaintance. When *FHM*'s editor emailed me to say that Professor Green wanted my number, I thought he was kidding, but Stephen called a few hours later. That was in November 2011 and by January we were a couple.

I moved in with him a year later and he proposed shortly after. It was a total surprise. Stephen said that he had to go Paris for a meeting with a designer and suggested that I go along too. I didn't suspect anything, even when I discovered that the 'cheap' hotel he'd said we were staying in turned out to be my favourite place, Hôtel Costes, because he was on the phone all the time to his agent discussing his meeting – which turned out to be just part of this elaborate plot to surprise me. He asked me to marry him over dinner that evening. The first thing I said was, 'Have you asked my dad?' (He had, two weeks earlier.) Looking back, I feel a bit sorry for Stephen because I spent the rest of the evening calling my family and friends. I don't think I ate anything!

I loved planning the wedding. We chose Babington House in Somerset because it's near to where I grew up and I wanted a proper, romantic country wedding. My dad and I had made a pact that we'd be strong for each other but, on the day, we totally failed; we were both crying as we walked down the aisle. Stephen says that the first thing he noticed when he saw me was that I had snot on my face!

It was getting engaged to Stephen that actually got me into fitness. I hated sport at school but I've always been slim, so I didn't think I really needed to work out. However, a combination of nights out drinking, sugar-laden food and takeaways was beginning to give me a muffin top and a double chin, which is not a good look for your wedding day! I started seeing Stephen's trainer. He did this test to check my body-fat percentage (basically, he pinched the skin on my cheek, back, stomach, bum, hip and thigh) and it came out at 27 per cent; 18–25 per cent is considered healthy and 32 per cent is obese, so I was definitely 'skinny fat'. In other words, although I was slim, I was metabolically fat and therefore at risk of developing exactly the same medical problems – high blood pressure, diabetes, etc. – as a visibly fat person. That was certainly a surprise! I began a fitness routine designed to burn fat and, because there's not much point in working out hard if you're eating the wrong things, I changed my diet too.

It's tempting to think that you can eat whatever you like when you're burning off lots of calories in the gym, but if you eat a chocolate bar before you train, all you do in the session is burn off the chocolate bar; you won't make any difference to your body fat or muscle tone. Eating well, i.e. making sure that you get the right balance of protein, fat and carbohydrate, gives you the energy you need to train and helps to convert fat into lean muscle. I'd be lying if I said I found it easy – I didn't – but I did start seeing results quite quickly and that spurred me on. By the time the wedding came round four months later, I had lost 10 per cent body fat; 17 per cent body fat is good if you're physically fit and work out often.

Exercise is quite addictive – the fitter you get, the better you feel – but a big reason why I keep at it is because it means that I don't have to diet. My metabolism isn't as fast as it was in my teens and eating has always been a major part of my life, so I need to keep active. I have quite extreme tastes in food. I generally prefer rich, savoury flavours but when I do eat sweet things, I really go for it and I find it hard to resist a slice of cake. I guess a fondness for sweet things is hardly surprising given that it was the Mackintoshes who invented Quality Street.

My great-great grandpa, John Mackintosh, was known as the 'toffee king' because he revolutionised the way we think about toffee. He was born in Lancashire in 1868 and got married in 1890. He and his wife Violet then opened a small shop in Halifax and my great-great granny worked on a recipe combining hard, brittle toffee with soft, American-style caramel. No one had ever done that before and people loved it. By 1895 they had set up a factory, and Mackintosh Ltd was formed four years later. Quality Street was created in 1936.

My dad remembers being taken on tours of the factory that sound just like the 'Toot Sweet' scene from *Chitty Chitty Bang Bang*. By the time I was born, the company had been sold, so I'm not an heiress, despite what the papers say. However, I am very proud that Quality Street is part of my heritage. My parents have a huge collection of vintage Quality Street tins and we named each table at my wedding after a different sweet from the range. Ours was Toffee Penny.

A love of food and cooking seems to be a family trait. My parents owned and ran a delicatessen, Mackintosh of Marlborough, and Mum used to let me help out in the kitchen buttering bread for the sandwiches and making Parmesan biscuits. Everyone was always amazed by my appetite – I'd ask for a cooked breakfast and then have

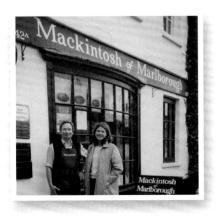

a massive bowl of pasta for lunch – but although I ate a lot (and I still do), I've never been a great one for junk food. But of course my diet took a nosedive when I first left home to move to London. Too much partying leads to bad food choices and unhealthy habits (pizza in bed!), so when I started exercising, I made a decision to look at what I was putting into my body too.

And now here I am in my mid-twenties. Like so many people, I don't know exactly what I'll be doing work-wise ten years from now, but I'm enjoying my life and I'm finally at ease with myself. It's not always great being recognised (I don't look my best when I'm popping out for a carton of almond milk at 7 a.m. on a rainy morning!), but one of the things I do love about being in the public eye is having people stop me to say how they've been inspired by something I've said or done. That's so flattering and I know just what they mean because I find other people's diet, fitness and beauty regimes great sources of inspiration too. I've met and worked with some fantastic personal trainers, nutritionists, fashion designers and make-up artists over the last few years and they've taught me so much and helped me to get in shape, inside and out. Stephen's trainer, Richard Marsh, and Russell Bateman of the Skinny Bitch Collective, for example, have shown me what my body is capable of and has helped me turn that excess body fat into muscle, while my friend and nutritionist Madeleine Shaw has helped me totally rethink my approach to eating. The things I have learned from them all has given me a sense of control, because now I know what to do if I start to feel that my jeans are becoming too tight, or if my skin has a freak-out. And that's why I wanted to write this book. I wanted to consolidate all the things I've learned and to pass them on. I'm not saying that this is the only way, or even the best way, to look after yourself; it's just what works for me.

I've called the book *Made* because I wanted to dispel the myth that getting to this point has been easy. It's true that I haven't ever been fat, but I have been uneasy in my body. (I used to dream of having a boob job – one of the most embarrassing moments of my adolescence was when the cotton wool I'd stuffed my bra with fell out in front of everyone at summer camp.) I have been lucky, but making a body I am happy with has taken hard work. And maintaining it is hard work too. I do it partly because keeping in shape is important for my job, of course, but I would stick to this regime anyway because it's a way of living that makes me feel good.

The book is divided into four sections – 'Style', 'Beauty', 'Food' and 'Fitness'. Each one contains lots of simple tips and ideas based on my own experience. 'Food' is filled with delicious, fuss-free, healthy recipes, as well as some handy hints on beating a hangover. 'Fitness' covers my go-to classes, home workouts and nutrition. 'Style' is full of suggestions on how to look great everywhere, from a tropical beach to a muddy festival field, and 'Beauty' is crammed with tips to help you make the most of what you've got. Not everything here will work for you, but I hope you'll give some of the ideas a try, and if something in these pages helps you find the best way of looking and feeling good, *Made* will have done its job. And if it tells you a few things you didn't know and makes you laugh too, then I'll be happy.

Love,

Millie

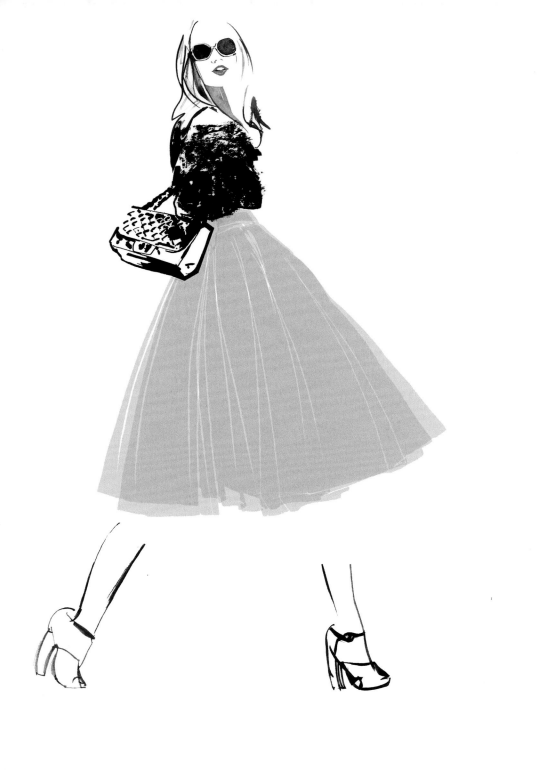

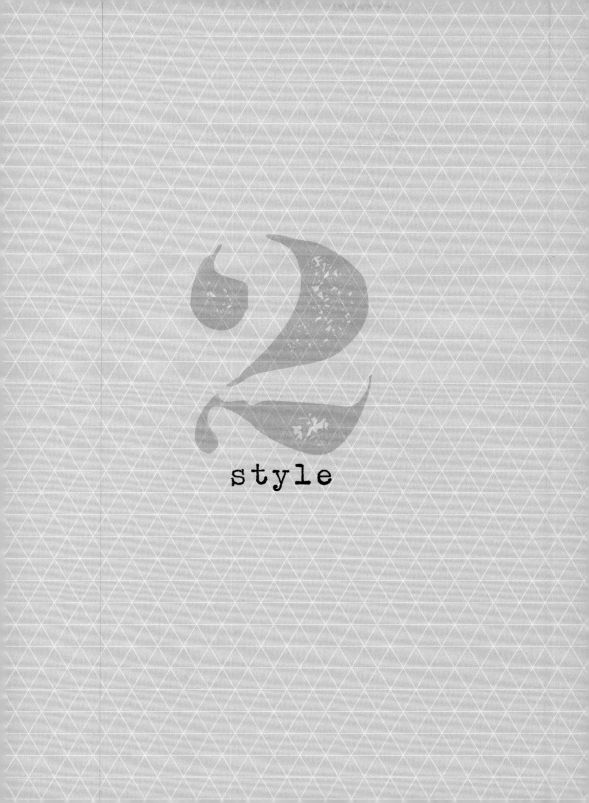

style

For me, fashion is about having fun. As a child, I wasn't remotely interested in wearing fashionable clothing, but I always loved dressing up, and by the age of ten I was making my own clothes. These mostly consisted of long, tube-shaped skirts with elasticated waists made from strange remnants (I remember one covered in dancing cats), but I thought they were great. Later I made a collection of baby-doll negligées as part of my BTEC diploma. They were really popular with my friends, so after I left school, I started making them in different fabrics and selling them as summer dresses.

Like most teenagers, I experimented with lots of different looks. At around 14, I thought a denim mini skirt worn with cowboy boots, a shirt with the collar up and backcombed hair was the height of cool. And then there was my Miss Sixty jeans and Ralph Lauren shirt obsession …

I buy things that make me feel like me: it's more about tailoring and timelessness than the latest look

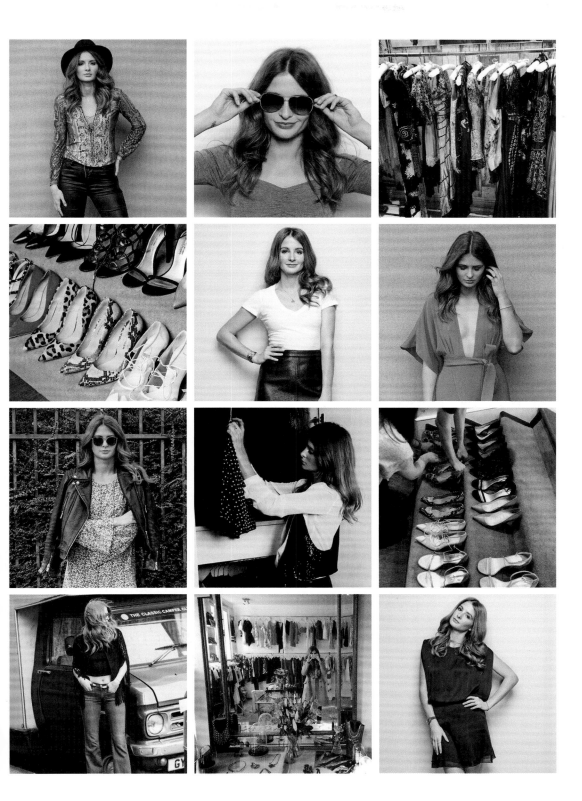

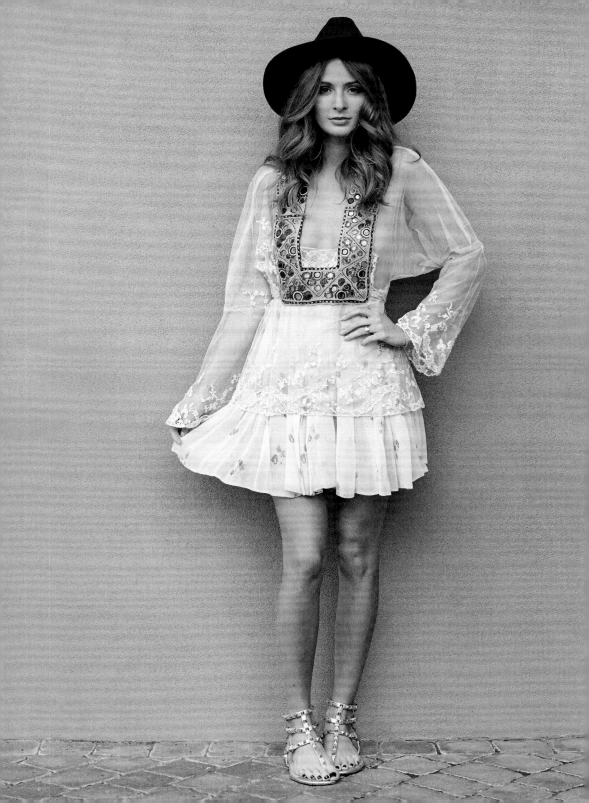

These days I buy rather than make my own clothes (my creativity goes into devising pieces for my fashion line – I let the professionals do the sewing) and I try to go for classic items that I can see myself still wanting to wear in ten years' time. I do keep track of fashion, of course, and I love the shows, but I don't shop on the basis of passing trends. I buy things that make me feel like me: it's more about tailoring and timelessness than the latest look – I am totally fixated on finding the perfectly cut black blazer, for instance. But the dressing-up thing hasn't gone away either. I'm drawn to vintage, boho styles and anything with a slightly gypsy, pirate, princess feel. I guess you can see the roots of that in those early, homemade clothes.

This section is not a definitive guide to fashion. You won't find information on body shapes or the best colours for certain skin tones, and you won't find a list of dos and don'ts either, because when it comes to clothes, I definitely don't believe in rules. (It's meant to be fun, remember?) What you will find are lots of details about my style and how I put my 'signature looks' together, an address book of brilliant shops, and some advice about dressing for festivals, holidays and special events based on my own personal experience. Oh, and because this is about my look, there's quite a lot about ankle boots, hats and over-sized cat-eye sunglasses too. Enjoy!

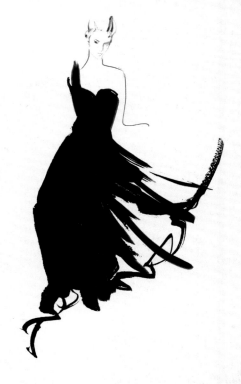

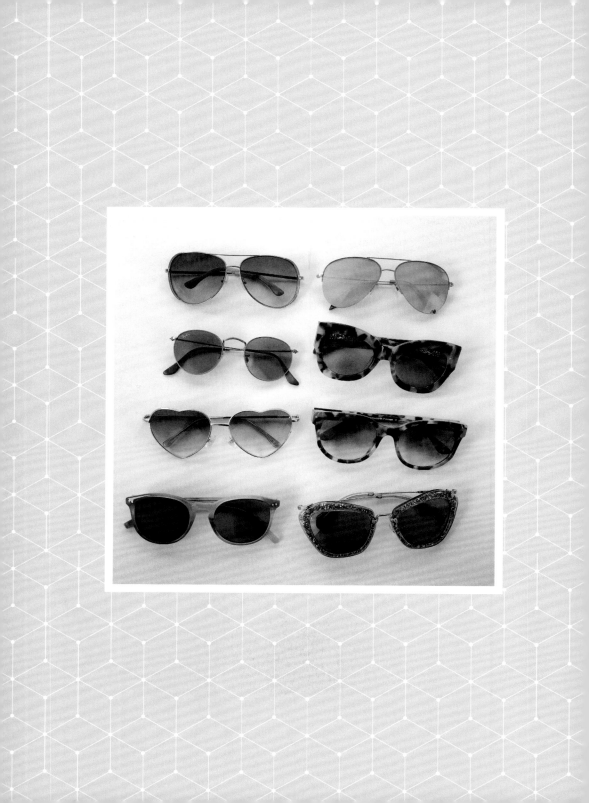

WARDROBE ESSENTIALS

Open my wardrobe and you'll find lots of fabulous, crazy things that wouldn't look out of place in a dressing-up box. However, in among the beaded jackets, the faux-fur stoles and vintage sunglasses, there are also lots of simple, quiet basics. They might not look that exciting on the hanger but these are the go-to pieces that make the other stuff work. Without them, the dressing-up things would be just that: dressing up.

Here is my list of essentials – buy the best you can afford because these are the clothes that you will wear day in, day out. I like to think in terms of cost per wear – if you wear that budget-busting jacket for the next decade, then it will have been a worthwhile investment.

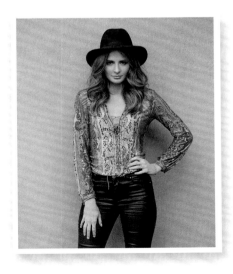

my key wardrobe items

★ Hero jeans in blue, black and grey – I like skinny ones with a high waistband that stops just above my hip bone.

★ Leather trousers.

★ Denim shorts.

★ Fine knitwear – much more flattering than bulky sweaters and you can layer them for warmth.

★ Good-quality cotton T-shirts in black, white, grey and navy.

★ Base layers in a variety of colours and weights for layering under knitwear.

★ Tailored white shirt with a collar.

★ Cotton blouses in white and cream.

★ Silk blouses in black and white.

★ Denim shirt.

★ A-line skirts in various lengths.

★ Little black dress (at least one!).

★ Daytime maxi dresses – one for each season.

★ Blazers – one dark, one cream. Make sure that each fits neatly across your shoulders.

★ Leather jacket.

★ Winter coat.

★ Ankle boots in black and tan.

★ Heels you can walk in – I like a heel with a platform at the front.

★ Strappy, nude sandals with a heel.

★ Platform sandals – great with flares or a mini dress.

★ Some really flattering swimwear.

★ Tote bag with room for everything.

★ Evening bag with a chain – just tuck the chain in if you want to use it as a clutch.

★ A piece of simple jewellery you can wear every day.

★ A piece of statement jewellery for special occasions.

UNDERWEAR

Underwear needs thinking about. It has to fit properly – nothing wrecks an outfit more than a VPL or ill-judged bra – and be in a colour that's appropriate for whatever you're wearing on top. Visible underwear can be a good look, but if you are going down that path, choose both the underwear and the occasion very carefully …

BRAS: I really do recommend going for a professional bra fitting. You need seamless, nude pieces for wearing under light-coloured clothes and a variety of bra shapes to suit different necklines. Nipple stickers, boob tape and stick-on bras are all good if you're not wearing a bra.

PANTS: Stock up on lots of different shapes, from thongs to boy shorts, and don't be afraid of Spanx: whatever your size, they can give you curves in all the right places and create a lovely smooth line under tight dresses.

SLIPS: I also have a few slips for wearing under sheer dresses. It is a good idea to have both a black and a nude version, and also to have them in a few different lengths.

HOSIERY: I still have nightmares about my fishnet tights days … Now my hosiery wardrobe contains lots of good-quality black tights ranging in thickness from sheer to opaque. I'm not into patterned tights (or colours), but I do like sheer black tights embellished with tiny polka dots. I also have several pairs of over-the-knee socks to wear with dresses and ankle socks to wear with skirts.

SHOES

Ankle boots are my daily staple. I own several pairs in black and tan, and the ones I live in most have a three-inch, chunky heel that is easy to walk in and flatters my feet. I also have some coloured ones, which are great with jeans. I'm a big fan of over-the-knee boots too – a pair of suede ones will bring just the right hint of sex appeal to a toned-down outfit.

I like a pointed heel, which draws the eye down so your legs seem longer. I do have rather a lot of heels, but the ones I couldn't do without are in black, both matt and patent, nude (perfect for when you want your dress to make the statement) – and to complement floaty, summer dresses), red and leopard print. There's nothing like a printed heel to spice up a simple outfit.

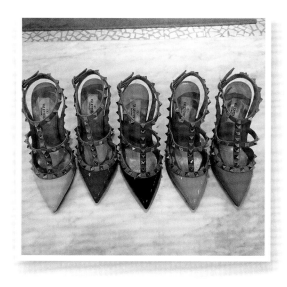

GOOD TO GO

Once you're set up, you can start having fun. (For how I team up these essentials to create my 'signature looks', see pages 44–51.) I do sometimes go to vintage stores and charity shops for original 1960s and 1970s designs, but I am careful not to overdo it, because I don't want to look like I'm in fancy dress. For me, one original piece in an outfit is enough.

a note on shopping

I am a spontaneous shopper and I love going with friends, but I have to admit that it's not always the most sensible approach as they can encourage you to buy clothes you don't really need or want. These are the things I try to remember to ask myself when I'm standing in the changing room:

★ Does it fit? We've all been there – so desperate for a certain dress that we'll convince ourselves that the only one left is the right size. Don't do it; ill-fitting clothes are never a good look.

★ Does it do my figure justice?

★ Am I willing to look after it? Read the care instructions before you buy the garment, so you know what you're letting yourself in for.

★ Do I already own something identical?

★ Do I wear it or does it wear me?

★ Will I want to wear it again? If it's a bargain, then it might not matter if you wear it only once or twice, but if you're investing, it needs to be something you'll want to hang on to.

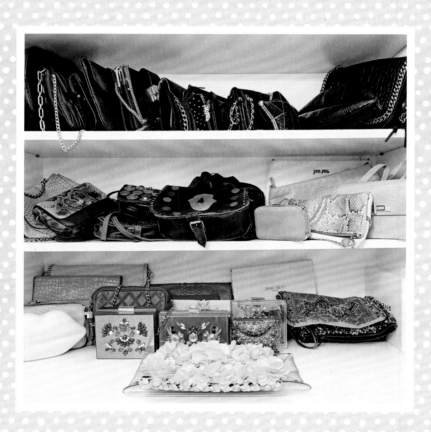

ACCESSORIES

Accessories are a great way of adding personality to a basic wardrobe. For example, classic jeans and a turtleneck sweater start to feel like me when paired with a pair of colourful heels, a belt with a gorgeous buckle and a hat. Here are my go-to essentials.

BAGS

Bags are a great way to change the look of an outfit. I do own a pretty large collection, but that's because I'd rather have different options than the latest 'It' bag (I hate owning the same thing as everyone else). As well as my essential tote and evening clutch, I also have casual bags for running errands and shoulder bags I can wear across my body when I might have other things to carry. (They're great for taking on shopping sprees when you need your hands free.) These days, I do quite like to co-ordinate my bag with my shoes or a hat, but not in too obvious a way; I might pick up the colour of my shoes in a ribbon on my hat, or reflect the gun-metal studs on my leather jacket with a silver zip on my bag. Details like this really pull a look together.

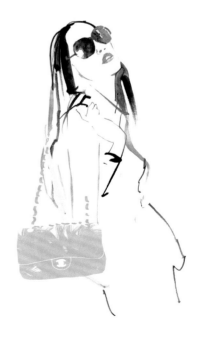

HATS

Hats have been a staple part of my wardrobe ever since I picked up my dad's fedora at the age of 16. They are a brilliant way to jazz up an outfit and finish off a look – I like to match a detail on the brim with the trim on a dress, for example, and I'll often team a monochrome outfit with a coloured hat.

SUNGLASSES

These are another obsession. Nanny Felicity always wore really wild ones and I think I've inherited the sunglasses gene. At the last count, I had ten pairs and I match them with my outfits (tortoiseshell frames look great with a tan bag, for instance) and my mood: aviators for a relaxed look; fun, coloured ones for summer festivals; and big, round ones when I want to look all Hollywood movie star – or simply need to hide baggy eyes. I don't wear them all the time, but in my book sunnies are definitely not just for summer.

Hats and sunglasses are an obsession: they reinvent any outfit and rescue me on the days when I don't feel at my best

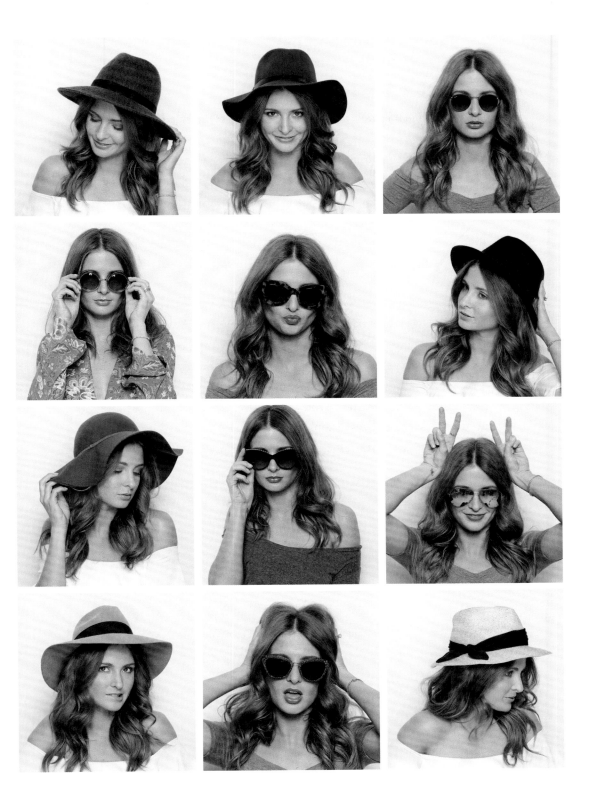

JEWELLERY

I like to combine gold and silver jewellery and my dressing table is home to mix of signature items like my M pendant, a few statement pieces for big nights out and lots and lots of jingly-jangly costume jewellery for holidays and festivals.

I had my ears pierced when I was about 12, but I don't wear earrings much these days – although I do like an ear cuff. This just slides onto one ear and makes you look as though you have multiple piercings. I quite like big hoops as well, although I would advise against wearing heavy earrings too often as they stretch your earlobes – not a good look!

Jewellery is such a personal thing, but I think less is more. When I'm going out for the evening, I either wear a statement necklace or statement earrings – never both at the same time. A gorgeous necklace will draw attention to your cleavage; earrings to your head.

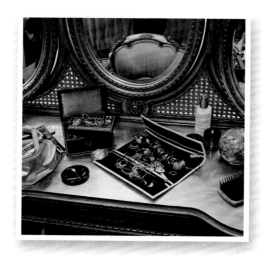

PUTTING IT TOGETHER

A collection of well-chosen accessories will also stretch your wardrobe to suit the occasion. These pictures show how you can transform three staple dresses from dressed-down cool to cocktail chic.

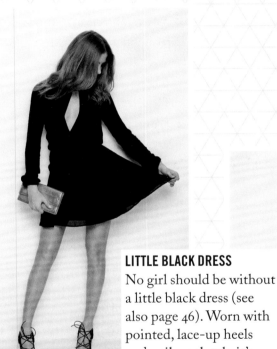

LITTLE BLACK DRESS
No girl should be without a little black dress (see also page 46). Worn with pointed, lace-up heels and a silver clutch, it's chic and sophisticated enough for date nights and cocktail parties; paired with over-the-knee boots, a belt and a hat, it's sassy and cool.

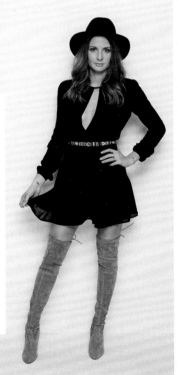

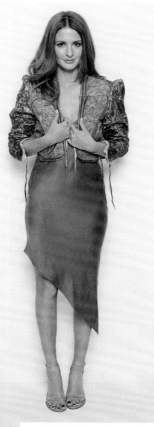

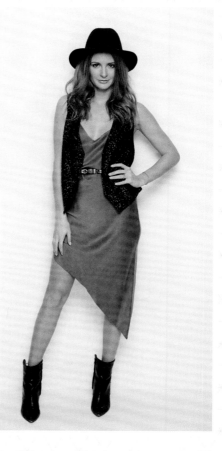

BIAS-CUT SLIP DRESS

This is a very simple shape
that can be styled up with
a gorgeous cropped jacket
(a short jacket draws attention
to your waist) for a special
occasion, or given a casual
boho vibe simply by swapping
the jacket for a sequinned
waistcoat and adding a thin
belt, hat and ankle boots.

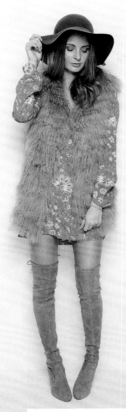

PRINTED DRESS

I love pretty printed dresses like this and find them really versatile. Add a fluffy gilet, a floppy hat and a pair of over-the-knee boots and you're ready for a festival or casual summer party, but with nothing more than simple sandals and a pair of sunnies, the same dress becomes a gorgeous beach cover-up.

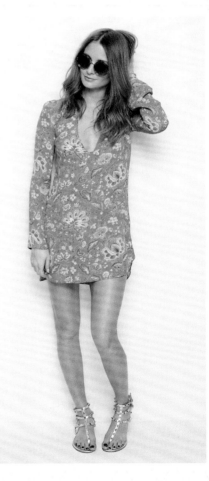

MILLIE'S SIGNATURE LOOKS

PERFECT-FIT CASUAL JEANS & CLASSIC T-SHIRT

Flared, skinny, boyfriend, bootcut – finding the perfect pair of jeans takes time and really you just have to go and try them on. Jeans are a classic, so don't be too swayed by current trends – choose the shape that best suits your figure. I like skinny ones that sit just above my hip bone.

No wardrobe is complete without a collection of good-quality T-shirts in classic plain colours (white, black, grey). I like cotton ones with a bit of stretch and a flattering V or deep scoop neck. If I'm just knocking about at home, then I'll finish this look off with a pair of ankle boots, but if I want to pep it up a bit, I'll go for a heel.

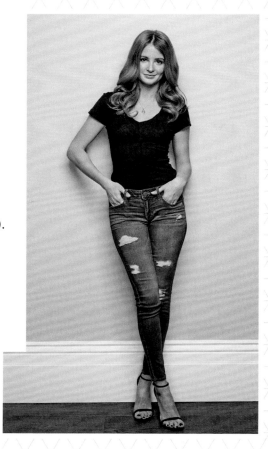

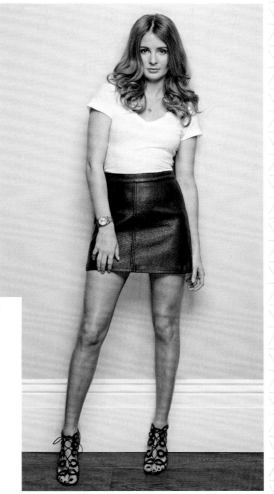

A-LINE MINI SKIRT

I've been a mini-skirt girl even since my granny bought me my first one when I was 13. It was literally a belt with a bit of fabric attached to it, but I remember her saying, 'If you've got it, flaunt it, honey; show off those pins!'

This leather mini is a wardrobe staple and a real favourite for a date night. In winter, I team it with sheer, polka-dot tights, thick knitwear and over-the-knee boots, while for a dressed-down summer look, I'll wear it with a simple V-neck T-shirt and a pair of high, sophisticated heels. I like the A-line shape because it skims over my hips.

BLACK JEANS & BLAZER

Banish all thoughts of shapeless school jackets: a tailored blazer is cool and sophisticated and will turn a look from casual to smart in an instant. For me, a blazer means business, so this is my go-to, fail-safe look for meetings. Wearing it undone and pulling the sleeves up slightly gives it a more relaxed feel.

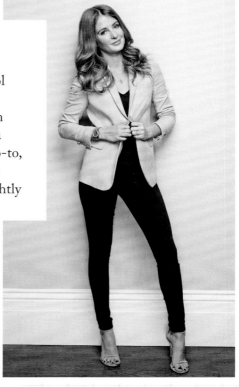

LITTLE BLACK DRESS

The point of a LBD is that you can just pull it out of the wardrobe, whack on some heels, do a quick revamp of your hair and make-up, and you're good to go. This silk dress, which I bought from Acne in a sale, has seen me through a few date nights. It's short and has that A-line shape that I love, but the high neckline balances out the hem.

JEANS, LEATHER JACKET, BIKER BOOTS & SCARF

This is the casual uniform that I reach for when I have no time to plan an outfit – the sort of thing I'll stuff in my gym bag if I have to go on somewhere after a workout. Leather jackets are fantastically versatile, toughening up a pretty summer tea dress or dressing down a smart maxi frock. They look great with jeans, but don't be tempted to wear one with leather trousers unless you really want to look like a biker!

The black and white print scarf around my neck adds some feminine softness, which is balanced by the biker boots. I like these contrasts – I am quite a girly girl, but I never want to look prissy.

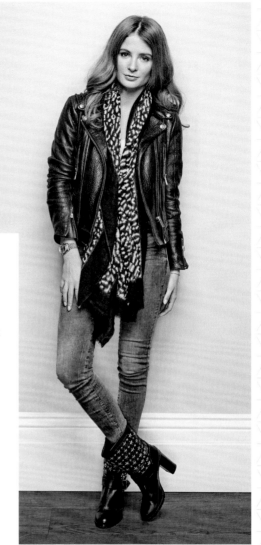

LEATHER LEGGINGS & SILK BLOUSE

I remember seeing some leather trousers in a shop when I was about ten and thinking how awful they were. Somewhere along the line I changed my mind and now they are a key part of my wardrobe. I love the way they can take me from day to evening depending on what I pair them with. Worn with some knitwear or a crisp shirt like this one, they're just right for a day at work, but teamed with a sheer blouse, they're super-sexy for a night out.

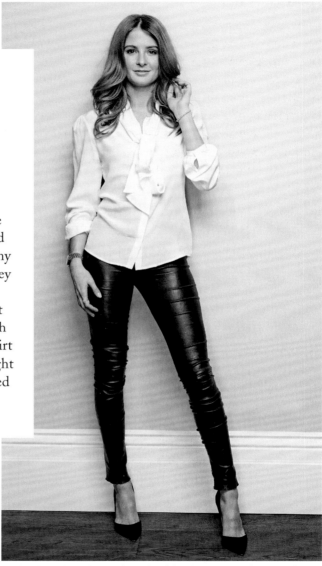

DAY DRESS & KNEE-HIGH BOOTS

I love easy dresses that I can just pull out and throw on. This one is really versatile – worn like this with over-the-knee boots, it's quite cool and cheeky (the demureness of the dress is balanced by that glimpse of thigh between the bottom of the hem and the top of the boot), but worn with nude ankle strap sandals, it would be perfect for a family party in the summer. I even wore it to London Fashion Week once, teamed with a big coat and biker boots.

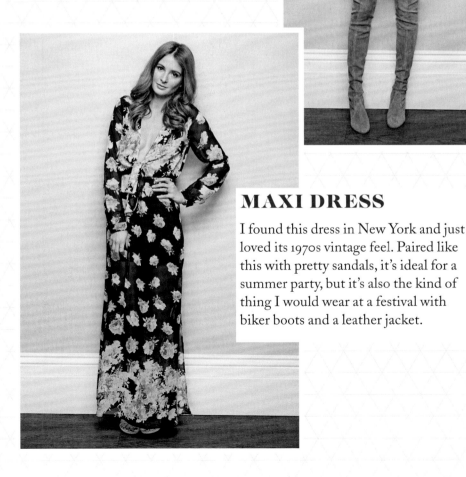

MAXI DRESS

I found this dress in New York and just loved its 1970s vintage feel. Paired like this with pretty sandals, it's ideal for a summer party, but it's also the kind of thing I would wear at a festival with biker boots and a leather jacket.

SHORT-SLEEVED POLO WITH A-LINE SUEDE SKIRT

I found this A-line skirt in M&S – it's a classic, flattering shape. Teamed with this short-sleeved polo top, it has a great 1970s vibe, while the heels bring the look right up to date.

SHIFT DRESS WITH CROCHET DETAIL & LONG BOOTS

This dress is from my own collection and is really easy to wear. The crochet detail gives it a retro feel without making it seem like fancy dress. Worn like this with long suede boots and a leather jacket, it's a perfect look for early spring.

FLARED JEANS, CROPPED VEST & SUEDE TASSEL JACKET

Flared jeans are so flattering. Worn like this, with a floaty tasselled jacket from my own collection and a pair of heart-shaped glasses, they are pure vintage cool and perfect for a festival.

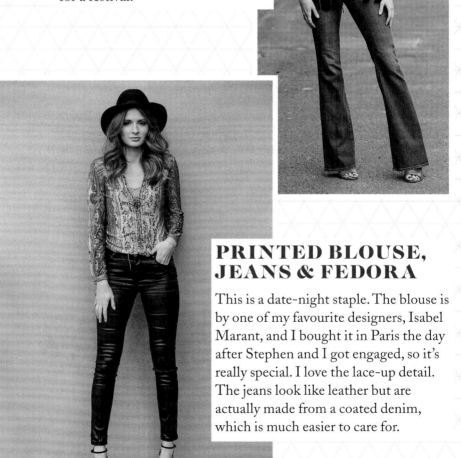

PRINTED BLOUSE, JEANS & FEDORA

This is a date-night staple. The blouse is by one of my favourite designers, Isabel Marant, and I bought it in Paris the day after Stephen and I got engaged, so it's really special. I love the lace-up detail. The jeans look like leather but are actually made from a coated denim, which is much easier to care for.

LOOKING YOUR BEST

Stylists are experts when it comes to making people look great. These are the wonderful Angie Smith's top figure-flattering tips:

#1

Shoes in a tone closest to you skin colour will make your legs look super-long.

#2

Elongate the lower half of your figure by faking the point of your waist. A belt, high-waisted trousers or skirt worn at the smallest and highest point of your waist are all perfect for this.

#3

Tuck your shirt into your trousers at the front to give you longer legs and a slimmer waistline.

#4

Always wear dark tones on the parts of your figure that you want to draw the eye away from and lighter hues on the parts you want to draw the eye towards. Flattering your figure is all about drawing attention to your best assets!

#5

To keep limbs and other parts of your body looking long, avoid contrasting lines that will chop them in two visually – think heels with ankle straps, clothes with horizontal stripes, dark thick bangles, chokers, dark nail varnish.

#6

Work out your perfect hem length and stick to it – it's usually either the point at which your thighs go in above the knee or that bit after your knee but before your calf curves out.

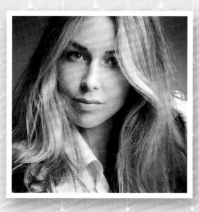

#7

The best way to find out what suits your shape is to work out your figure type and then dress against it. For example, girls with curves look great in more tailored shapes to give their body definition, while girls with a more athletic physique look better in layers and can experiment with textured fabrics and softer styles.

#8

You don't have to always belt your waist or wear fitted clothes to make yourself look slimmer. You might have an 'apple' shape with slender arms and legs, but by wearing A-line or boxy skirts, you can trick the eye to assume that because you have slim arms and legs your waistline must be the same!

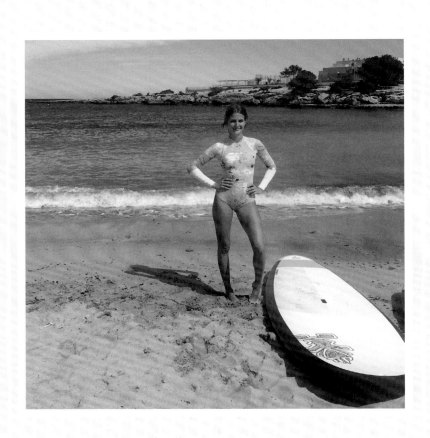

HOLIDAYS

The secret to a successful holiday wardrobe is planning. Time spent working out your outfits before you go will both ensure you look great and don't exceed your luggage allowance.

ON THE PLANE

It's important to be comfortable on a flight and you also need to be prepared for the change in temperature on board. Layers are the key. I usually opt for a maxi dress with a cardie, or jeans, T-shirt and a sweater. I'll also take an over-sized cashmere wrap in case I get cold.

Shoes need to be comfortable, so I'll go for sandals or espadrille wedges and I'll bring a hat. This not only saves space, but it also covers up post-flight hair disasters. Sunglasses are a must because flying gives me puffy eyes. (I never travel without an eye mask in my hand luggage.) I use my beach bag as my airport bag to save space.

BEACH HOLIDAYS

Beach holidays are a chance to go to town with gorgeous textures, bright colours and floaty fabrics. I start by spreading out all the clothes I want to take and sorting them into colour themes. I normally change my outfit twice a day on holiday – daytime beach wear and a look for the evening. Daytime means beach cover-ups like sarongs, denim hot pants, wrap skirts, kimonos and kaftans – and lots of swimwear. High-waisted bikini bottoms are the best shape for me, teamed with a top with a bit of lift. I like to take two different styles to wear each day (yes, two a day!) so I don't get a solid tan line. I use the colour of my swimwear as inspiration for the beach cover-ups. (Keep in mind that different countries have different dress codes – if going to Dubai or Morocco, you will need to cover up in public.)

I will also take a couple of summery maxi dresses for sightseeing, paired with espadrille wedges, a big hat and a cross-body bag to leave my hands free for any spontaneous purchases.

For the evenings, I'll pack something that looks great with tanned skin, like a red silk playsuit or a white maxi dress – lovely for more dressed-up occasions. If I'm going to Ibiza, I'll go for a more festival, party feel and focus on pieces with lots bright colour, bold prints and interesting embellishments.

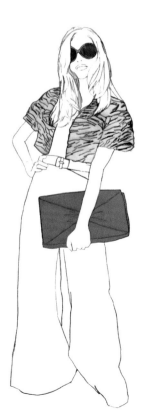

CITY BREAKS

I like to dress in the style of the city I'm visiting, so if it's Paris then I go for monochrome – lots of stripy T-shirts, my black beret, cat-eye sunnies and things with bows on. Or I'll take inspiration from one of that country's top designers: Acne for a trip to Sweden, for example. I start by choosing my key pieces and then look at the colour scheme I'm making and work from that. For example, black and white with hints of aubergine, with a scarf and ankle boots in the same colour.

my city break packing list:

★ Casual jeans.

★ Smart leather trousers.

★ Favourite stripy top.

★ Lightweight jumpers.

★ Silk evening blouse in white or cream.

★ Little black dress.

★ Smart tailored blazer.

★ Coats – one for the day, one for evening.

★ Burberry mac.

★ Ankle boots with a chunky heel – city breaks mean a lot of walking, so comfort is vital. I never take new shoes – that's a sure route to blisters.

★ Over-the-knee boots.

★ Heels for evening.

★ Cross-body bag.

★ Travel tote bag.

★ Evening clutch bag.

★ Black sunnies.

★ Hat – black fedora to cover up any hair disasters.

★ I also make sure that I leave a little space for a few new buys. I like to collect pieces from the country I'm visiting to remind me of my trip and to embrace the fashion of a different, exciting culture.

I WILL ALSO BRING:

 # SHOES – good flat sandals are a must. I love gladiator sandals and I normally take two pairs, one black and one metallic, because they go with everything. Plus wedges and heeled sandals for evenings and some flip flops for the beach.

 # UNDERWEAR – a mix of nude seamless, summery pieces and bright colours to wear under sheer garments (see page 33 for tips on selecting underwear).

 # SLIPS TO SLEEP IN – lightweight pyjamas or a silky nightie in case there's air conditioning.

 # SUNGLASSES – I'm not one to take a single pair of sunnies; just like shoes, different sunglasses go with different outfits. I'll usually take one black, one tortoiseshell and one coloured pair. Oh, and a casual aviator and a cat-eye too, just in case.

 # HATS – not just because they look great, but because they protect my face and chest from the sun. No one likes a crêpey chest after all!

 # TRAVEL BAG – this usually doubles as my beach bag.

 # CLUTCH BAG for evenings.

 # JEWELLERY

 # GYM KIT, INCLUDING TRAINERS – I like to pack really colourful, matching shorts and sport bras for holiday workouts.

 # SNORKEL AND REEF SHOES

 # MAKE-UP BAG

 # WASH BAG

 # PASSPORT!

my packing tips

And once you have your outfits sorted, all that remains is to get them in your suitcase. Here are my top packing tips:

★ Roll items that crease easily.

★ Save space by packing hats upside down and filling them with bikinis, underwear and scarves. This helps hold their shape too.

★ Pack shoes with your toiletries, ideally in a separate case.

★ Use a rigid, waterproof case – it gives more protection than canvas and your clothes won't get as creased.

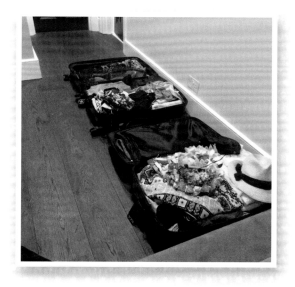

DATES

Obviously, you are going to want to look your best on a date, but you also want to be comfortable. Choose clothes that reflect your personality and make the most of your best assets. My legs are mine (thanks, Mum!), so I usually go short for a date, though for my first one with Stephen I wore red, wax-coated jeans, black knee-length boots, a leopard-print cardigan, buttoned to the top, and a black shearling coat. It was figure-hugging but I was completely covered up. As a teenager, I thought that less was more on a date, but these days I'd say it's better not to give too much away. I wouldn't do short and low cut, for example. You can be sexy in lots of subtle ways – show a bit of back, expose one shoulder, reveal a hint of cleavage.

Ideally, dates coincide with days when you're looking great, but if not, DO NOT DESPAIR! Clothes can work wonders – here are my top tips (learned from bitter experience!):

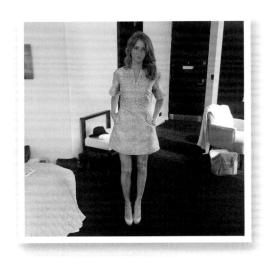

Wear something that's more colourful than you're feeling.

Adopt the look of a style icon who is cooler than you could ever hope to be – my go-to icons are Kate Moss and Alexa Chung.

Put on a pair of heels – a killer heel is guaranteed to make you walk with confidence. But do make sure you can actually walk in them … I once wore a pair of orange and blue leopard-print Brian Atwood heels for a night out with Stephen. I'd seen Cheryl Cole wearing them and had totally fallen in love, but they were so high that I couldn't walk and I had to ask a waiter to help me get to the loo!

Wear something you know has worked before.

Fake it: a padded bra, a pair of Spanx – whatever it takes to maximise or minimise those assets!

Remember, most guys don't really notice what you're wearing – they certainly won't spot whether your shoes match a detail on your bag. What they will notice is how confident you are, so wear something that makes you feel good.

If you're going to eat, you will spend most of the evening sitting at the table, so wear something that draws attention to your face.

And if the light levels are likely to be low, wear a necklace that brightens your skin.

PARTIES

How to dress depends on the party, of course, but if there is a dress code on the invitation, stick to it. Here are some pointers.

HOUSE PARTIES

If we're entertaining at home, I like to keep it casual so will probably go for jeans, a shirt and pair of heels (which I take off soon after everyone's arrived!). If we're going to a friend's place, then it will probably be a mini skirt, shirt and leather jacket. Plus a great pair of ankle boots.

THEMED PARTIES

I love fancy-dress parties as they are a chance to have fun. I usually work with what I have in my wardrobe (black leather leggings, over-the-knee boots and a black top is a fail-safe cat woman), then just buy a few funny accessories (like a tail and a cat woman mask).

COCKTAIL PARTIES

I usually go for my little black dress (see pages 42 and 46), a suit with shorts or a classic trouser suit. I'm a big fan of trouser suits – they look great with nothing underneath the jacket (stick the sides with body tape to avoid revealing too much) and a slightly flared trouser.

BLACK-TIE PARTIES

Black-tie parties are a chance to bring out that wow dress. I like to go full length – one of my favourite outfits is a long, halter-neck column dress with subtle stud detailing around the collar that really shows off my shoulders and is a good shape for a small bust. Or I might wear a tux with nothing underneath the jacket (don't forget the tape!).

I go to lots of events and sometimes I'm lucky enough to get to borrow a gorgeous frock, but you don't need to have lots of evening dresses. Invest in a simple maxi dress – something quite close-fitting with straps and a clean neckline, for example – and ring the changes with accessories. Try an embellished bolero jacket, a faux-fur stole, a pair of long gloves or a belt.

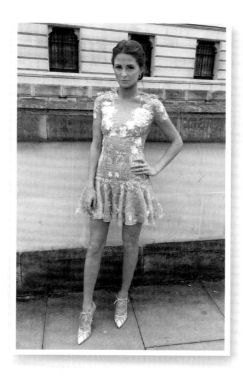

FESTIVALS

Packing for a festival reminds me of my childhood dressing-up box. I like to indulge my inner hippie, so I pull out everything I own that has tassels, sequins, beading or lace and often combine it all in one look. This is festival fashion, so anything goes. (Or almost anything – bum cheeks hanging out of denim cut-offs should definitely be prohibited, along with visible bras. You know who you are, girls!)

I pack for every season when I'm going to a British festival. If it's cold and damp (I don't go if it's pouring), I'll wear Wellies – I have a Matthew Williamson pair with feathers on them – ripped jeans, an army or leather jacket (you won't catch me in a plastic poncho!), and a fedora or a trilby.

On a hot, sunny day, I'll go for either a boho maxi dress or hot pants and a crop top with ankle boots, because you do need to protect your feet. I'm fond of a floral wreath on my head too. Whatever the weather, I pile on the jewellery – armfuls of bangles and long, beaded necklaces, and I never leave my tent without over-sized sunnies.

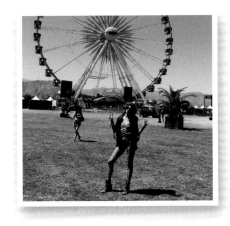

my essential festival packing list

★ Wellies and/or biker boots.

★ Converse or trainers.

★ Socks – to keep your feet warm and prevent Wellie blisters.

★ Ripped casual jeans – take enough pairs to wear two per day, especially if you are going to a festival in the UK.

★ Warm layers.

★ Faux fur or waterproof coat.

★ Hats – essential for bad weather and bad-hair days. Don't expect them to make it home again, though, so leave the designer ones behind.

★ Headdresses or floral headbands – wrong everywhere other than a festival or wedding, so enjoy!

★ Warm tracksuit to sleep in – this is one occasion where you can get away with a cashmere onesie and UGG boots …

★ Sunnies – the sun may not shine, but you will need to hide your hangover.

★ Cross-body bag to leave your hands free when walking around, dancing or navigating a Portaloo.

★ Make-up kit.

★ Wash bag containing earplugs, eye mask, hand sanitiser, paracetamol, Imodium, Berocca and Dioralyte.

★ Warm sleeping bag.

★ Tent.

★ Camping chair.

WEDDINGS

I absolutely loved choosing my dress. It was by Alice Temperley and
the moment I saw it and tried it on, I knew it was right because it was
exactly how I had always imagined I would look on my wedding day.
The dress had this timeless, slightly vintage look and made me feel
like a princess but without being a big meringue; it was really elegant
and sophisticated. I chose it quickly but I made lots of Pinterest
boards and did masses of research beforehand, so I had a good idea
of what I was looking for. There are whole books and magazines
dedicated to weddings, but here are just a few tips based on my
own experience:

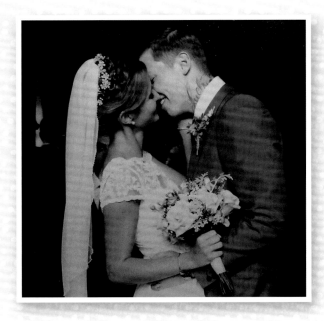

DO YOUR RESEARCH before you start making appointments –
it really does help to have an idea of what you want.

DON'T TAKE MORE THAN TWO PEOPLE WITH YOU. Too many different
opinions just gets confusing.

TRY THINGS ON – you need to see yourself in the dress.

WHEN YOU LOOK AT YOUR REFLECTION, ask yourself whether you
see you. You want to look like the best version of yourself on your
wedding day, not like a completely different person.

IS IT COMFORTABLE and do you feel secure? The last thing you want
to be worrying about is falling out of your dress.

DON'T WORRY TOO MUCH ABOUT EVERYTHING MATCHING. My
bridesmaids' dresses – inspired by the colour of some roses I was
given when I got engaged – did match each other, but I don't think
it's essential. In fact, having each bridesmaid in a different dress
can look lovely, especially if there's a big age range.

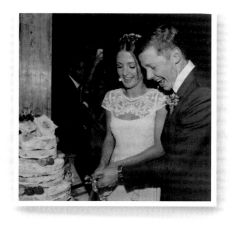

and a few tips for wedding guests

★ Don't wear white – that's the bride's privilege. And don't wear anything too sexy. I have a fuchsia-pink, mid-calf-length dress which I like for summer weddings.

★ Be respectful – this is a wedding, not a beach or a night club. If there's a party in the evening, think about changing or covering your shoulders for the ceremony. I went to a black-tie wedding in a long, floral-print, column-shaped dress once and just wore a little cardie over it for the ceremony.

★ Don't upstage the bride's mother!

★ If you decide to wear a hat, make sure it's not so large that it blocks the view for other people. I prefer just to wear a flower in my hair.

★ Always follow the dress code.

★ Don't wait to decide what you are going to wear until the weekend before; you will end up panic buying something you do not really want.

★ If you don't want (or can't afford) to buy a new dress ask a friend if you can borrow or swap one of your dresses with one of theirs. Another option is to use a hiring service; www.girlmeetsdress.com stocks a great selection.

★ If you are buying a new dress, make sure that you already have shoes and a bag that complement it. The last thing you want to do is to have to buy a brand new bag and shoes to match as well!

THE RACES

The rules are much slacker than they used to be, but I still like to acknowledge them and respect the traditions. For me, the perfect race-day outfit is a Victoria Beckham pencil-skirt dress (you can find similar style dresses on the high street), but a trouser suit worn with a blouse also makes a great statement. I always go for a soft colour or neutrals – nothing too garish – and stick to matt fabrics (this is daytime after all). And a hat is a must! Your shoes need to comfortable, so I'd wear a heeled sandal with a wedge at the front. Bag-wise, I'd go for a clutch with a strap so I could wear it over my shoulder if needs be.

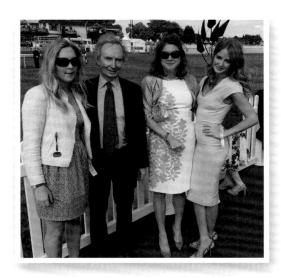

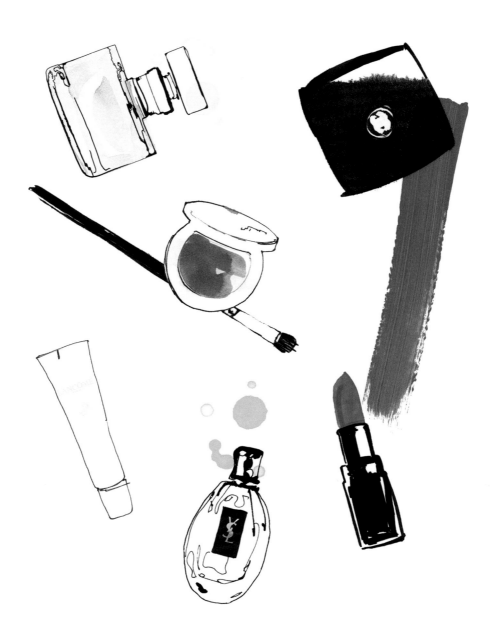

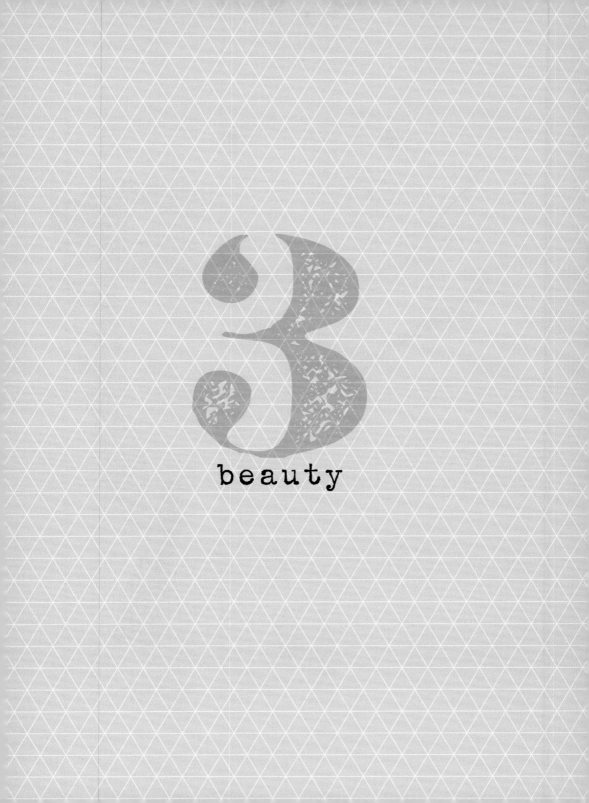

3

beauty

Beauty has been my thing ever since I discovered peel-off childrens nail varnish at the age of six. Mum bought it for me in a rare moment of weakness (she was in a hurry) after I threw a monumental strop in a toy shop in Marlborough. In the end, my precious purchase ended up all over the play room carpet because I left it on the floor with the lid off and our pug, Myrtle, promptly knocked it over, but when I first arrived home with that bottle of purple, glittery liquid, I was so excited that I couldn't speak.

A few years later, I managed to persuade my two grandmothers to start handing down their beauty cast-offs. There was foundation and blusher from chic Granny Jennifer (who was always perfectly golden brown with lovely wavy blonde hair) and from Dad's mum, the glamorous Nanny Felicity, there was a gorgeous Chanel eye-shadow palette and nail polish (telephone-box red and the real deal, yes!) and a Yves Saint Laurent perfume that was so strong that it nearly made me faint. I thought I had arrived.

*Make-up is there
to play with, to enhance
our best bits and to help
us express our differences
and individuality*

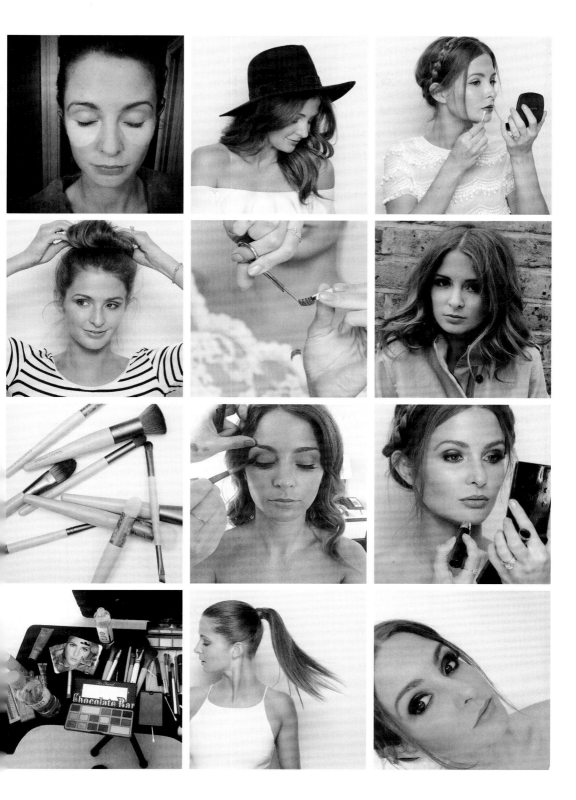

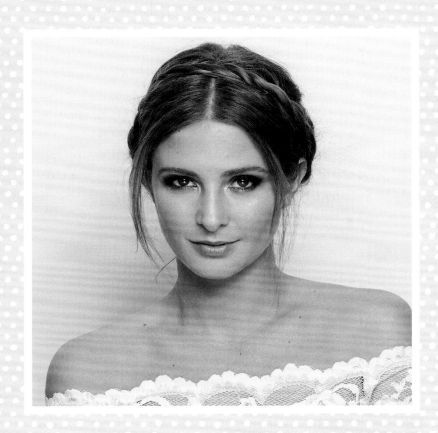

I soon realised that there was more to this stuff than expensive, tactile packaging and irresistible colours. Watching Mum get ready for parties taught me that make-up could be a power player. Every weekend there was a cocktail party, barbecue or theatre trip and I looked on, transfixed, as Everyday Mummy transformed herself into Evening Mummy by adding just a few small touches of make-up.

As I got older and began experimenting properly with make-up and other beauty products, I discovered that this enchanted ritual had a dual purpose. I found that people looked at me quite differently when I was wearing a sleek ponytail and a fierce red lip, rather than just stumbling out of the house with nothing on my face, and I also discovered that I got a powerful emotional charge by smoothing on a delicious face cream, taking an indulgent bath with a drop of my favourite essential oil or applying a coat of coral nail polish at the end of a bad day.

And so I came to realise that 'beauty' and make-up are not really about looking a particular way, or about this season's must-have shade or style; they're about discovering how to look and feel the best you can. There is no right or wrong way and no great need to conform. We are each born with a different face, skin, nose, lips and brow, and that's what makes us interesting. Make-up is there to play with, to enhance our best bits and to help us express our differences and individuality.

Most of what I know about make-up and beauty I taught myself – with the help of Mary Quant's book *Classic Make-up & Beauty*, Jemma Kidd's *Jemma Kidd Make-up Masterclass* and lots of issues of *Vogue*. (I tore out every shoot that make-up artist Charlotte Tilbury worked on, because I loved the way she could change a face but in a way that still allowed the model's features to come through.) I spent my teenage years experimenting on myself and my long-suffering family and friends. Makeovers became my speciality and at secondary school I was quite often asked to do people's make-up for the annual leavers' dance. I remember on one occasion doing wonderful gold eyes for a particular girl and then putting her false lashes on the wrong way round. I was too embarrassed to say anything and luckily she didn't seem to notice!

I have had some professional teaching too. I did a two-month course at the Glauca Rossi School of Make Up in west London when I first left school and I worked at Space NK before joining *Made in Chelsea*. Since then, I've done lots of TV and modelling, which has given me the chance to pick the brains of some super-talented make-up artists.

So as you can see, I am a lifelong beauty obsessive. It's an obsession that has left me with a bathroom full of bottles and a head full of information about skin care and make-up. This chapter is all about passing my best tips and ideas on to you.

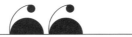

I wore this dressing gown
the morning of my wedding.
I wanted to be wearing something
beautiful even when I was
having my make-up done

FACE

Your face needs daily care and attention to keep it looking radiant.
Love your face and it will love you back – I promise.

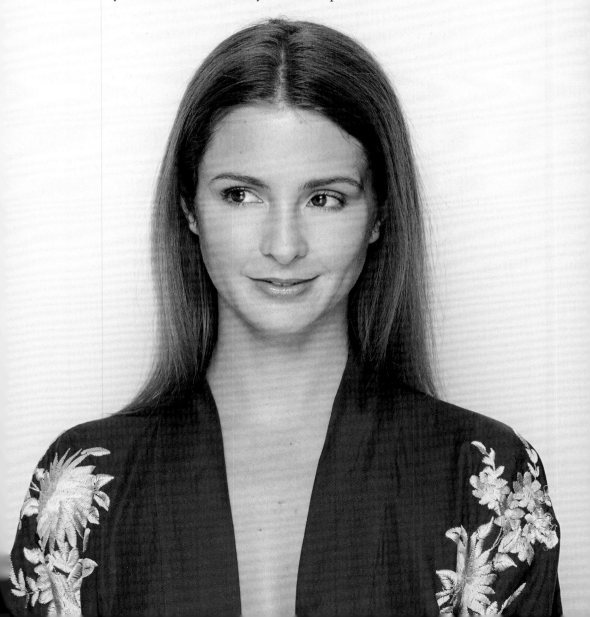

A NOTE ON SKIN TYPES

There are five basic skin types, although it is quite common to be more than one. Mine, for example, is a mix of combination and sensitive. Knowing your own skin type is important because it determines the type of products you use.

#1 DRY

The signs are flaky skin that looks and feels rough, fines lines and dullness. Your skin may also feel tight, especially after you've washed it. The good news is that you're unlikely to get spots.

#2 NORMAL

Characterised by barely-there pores, few imperfections and a natural radiance. If this is you, then you're very lucky!

#3 COMBINATION

This sort of skin is oily through the T-zone (forehead, nose, mouth area and chin) and dry elsewhere.

#4 OILY

If you can see enlarged pores and have a tendency to shine, then you have oily skin. This does mean that you are likely to suffer from blackheads, pimples and other blemishes, but on the plus side, your skin will age more slowly.

#5 SENSITIVE

The signs are redness, irritation, dryness and breakouts. This sort of skin needs careful handling.

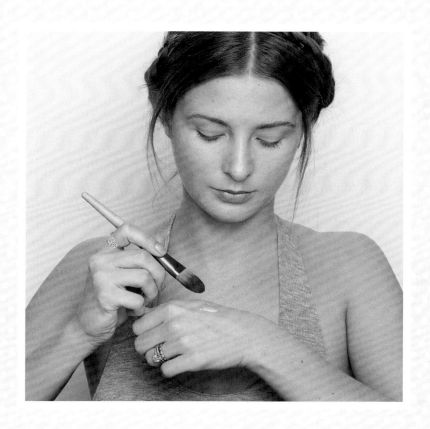

CARING FOR YOUR SKIN

I'm not into rules and regulations, but sometimes we all need to hear a few home truths. For me, this is the most important one: we girls can wear all the concealer, foundation and pressed powder in the world, but temporary make-up solutions don't last and don't make your skin look nearly as great as being happy and healthy. That's to say, exercising regularly, eating plenty of good, healthy things, sleeping lots and drinking loads of water are the very best things for feeling great and looking good too. Think of it as what you put in, you get out …

At school my long-suffering teachers were always talking about 'aims'. Whether it was a science experiment or an English essay, you always had to set them out before you got stuck in. So, following their example, here are my three 'aims' for good skin care:

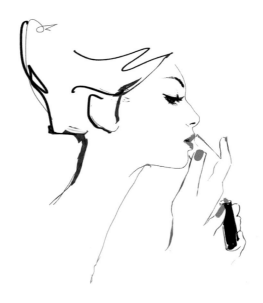

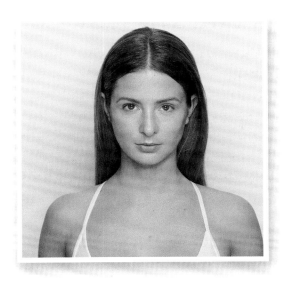

#1

Aim to protect your skin from environmental damage. Skin is delicate and sun, wind, pollution and even cigarette smoke will all cause harm.

#2

Aim to keep your skin well balanced – i.e. not too dehydrated in winter or too oily in summer. You may well need to alter your skin-care routine with the seasons.

#3

Aim to prevent premature ageing by using products containing antioxidants and by eating plenty of antioxidant-rich foods such as blueberries, broccoli and carrots.

However, even the best-fed, most well-rested skin needs a bit of help to look its absolute best. On the following pages is a guide to some of the products and practices that I consider to be essential.

CLEANSERS

Washing your face may sound like the easiest thing in the world, but in fact most people are terrible at cleansing, which can lead to all sorts of problems – mainly of the spotty variety. Until I started working at Space NK, I thought that slapping some cleanser haphazardly around my face for a few seconds before splashing it off with warm water was adequate. Now I know that cleansing your face, like brushing your teeth, should take about two minutes. It is primarily about getting rid of dirt and stale make-up, but think of it also as a luxurious and soothing little ritual that, if kept to, will improve your skin over time.

This is how you do it. (And I am forever grateful to a wise woman in the beauty industry who told me that if I changed nothing in my regime but followed these steps every night and morning, I would notice a difference in my skin. She was right.)

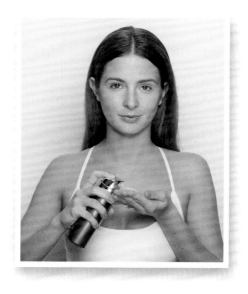

#1

Apply cleanser to dry skin with damp hands. The moisture on your fingers will improve the general spreadability and emulsification of the cleanser.

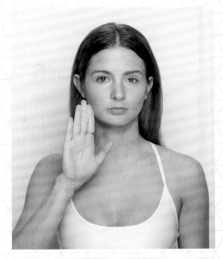

#2

Put a small amount of cleanser on your fingertips and place your hands, with your fingers pointing upwards, on either side of your nose.

#3

Starting at this centre point of your face, use small circular movements to massage the cleanser into your skin and spread slowly to the outer edges.

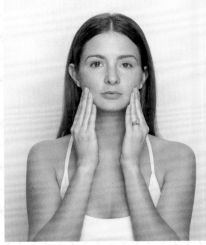

#4

Spend some time massaging the outer edges of your face and hairline as this is where all the lymph glands are and giving these some attention will aid lymphatic drainage and help make your face look more sculpted.

#5

Remove the cleanser with a warm flannel, face cloth or cotton wool.

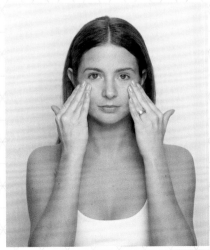

VARIOUS TYPES OF CLEANSER ARE AVAILABLE:

CLEANSING CREAM: Apply straight onto dry skin, massage in and remove with warm water on a cotton-wool pad or with some gentle, alcohol-free toner. Cream is soothing for sensitive skin and works well on drier or more mature skin.

CLEANSING WATER: This is water and cleanser in one, so it's great if you're in a hurry. (Before a night out, have some ready by your bed with a few cotton-wool pads.) Remember to start with your eyes, though, or you will be rubbing eye make-up all over your newly washed face.

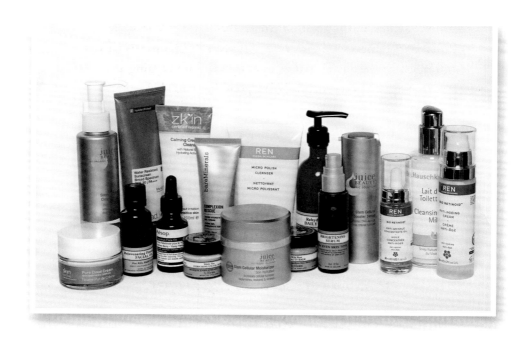

FOAMING CLEANSER: Use on wet skin, massage in and rinse off with water. Look for ones with a mild anti-bacterial ingredient if you have oily skin or with moisturising properties for dry skin.

EXFOLIATING CLEANSER: Exfoliation is extremely good for your face; it clears away dead cells so that the beneficial ingredients in your lotions and potions can penetrate your skin more easily, producing better results. Conveniently, removing the scummy dead cells also makes your face look glowy and fabulous. However, a little goes a long way. Strong and scratchy exfoliants can actually wound the surface of your skin, causing it to go into panic mode and produce a brand new layer. Long term, this process of wounding and healing leaves the skin looking thin and tired. Two or three times a week, I use an exfoliating cleanser with fruit or salicylic acid that gently dissolves dead skin cells without being abrasive. I massage the exfoliator into the areas of my face that need attention – usually my forehead, nose and chin. Do it gently: random tugging and over-enthusiastic scrubbing is NOT good for your skin.

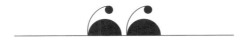

If you change nothing else in your regime apart from cleansing every night and morning, you will still notice a positive difference in your skin: this is worth doing properly

OIL-BASED CLEANSER: Apply straight onto dry skin, massage in and remove with a white muslin cloth – see 'Toners' below. (This will also gently exfoliate the skin. I have eight cloths and just bung them in the washing machine – without fabric conditioner because it changes the texture.) Oil-based cleansers are good for dehydrated skin, but contrary to what many people think, they are also suitable for oily and combination skin like mine because the oil in the product actually helps to remove oil in the skin.

TONERS: Toner is designed to remove cream cleanser and any final traces of make-up and dirt. Like many women, I learned the 'cleanse, tone, moisturise' mantra at a young age and followed it religiously. These days, however, unless I am having a nasty breakout of spots, I leave the tone stage out and simply remove oil-based cleanser with a white muslin cloth. (The microfibres in the fabric help to suck up the dirt and the whiteness makes it easy to see when your face is clean.) The reason I gave up toner is partly because lots of them contain harsh ingredients, such as alcohol, which irritate my skin and partly because it's not really necessary anyway since modern cleansers are designed to be washed away without leaving any residue. One thing I do use toner for, however, is to zap a nasty spot (see page 95 for details).

MOISTURISERS AND SERUMS: Both moisturisers and serums help to keep your skin looking and feeling hydrated, but they work in different ways. Serum sinks deeper into the skin, operating on the dermis, while moisturiser works on the surface, forming a layer that protects against the elements.

Different serums are directed at different aspects of skin care – some hydrate, some add brightness, some target signs of ageing – and you apply them before your moisturiser. They can be used on both your face and eyes, so you don't need separate products. I always use one containing hyaluronic acid, a substance that occurs naturally in the body and helps the skin to retain moisture and eliminate lines and wrinkles.

Moisturisers also come in many different varieties and the one you choose will depend on your own personal needs. Day moisturisers tend to be lighter. (Go for an oil-free one if you have oily skin, a hydrating one if your skin is dry. I like to use one with sun protection too.) Night-time moisturisers are rich and heavy, which is ideal for more mature skin but can be a bit too much for younger people. I prefer to use a facial oil at night – two or three drops pressed into my skin helps to plump up and rejuvenate my face.

Cleansing your face, like brushing your teeth, should take about two minutes

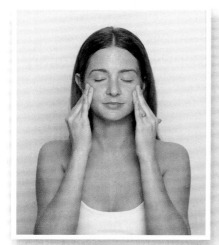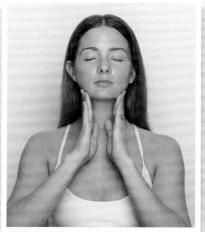

FACIAL MASSAGE

Take note, ladies: massage is as effective in the fight against signs of ageing as all those anti-ageing products. Basically, as we age our skin loses the ability to replenish lost cells, resulting in sagging skin and wrinkles. An hour of careful muscle manipulation will effectively act as a natural facelift, firming, calming and soothing the skin, leaving it restored to its beautiful best.

Obviously, if you do have the chance to indulge in a professional facial, then you should take it, but you can do a perfectly good face massage in the privacy of your own bathroom. Here's how to go about it and what areas to focus on:

FACIAL OIL: Before you start, you need to get yourself some good facial oil. This applies even if you have oily skin because serums disappear into the skin too quickly. Don't panic: the oil will balance rather than overload your skin.

SAGGING: Tight facial muscles equal smooth skin. Give them a regular workout by massaging your face using long, diagonal, upwards strokes. (Our facial muscles are arranged diagonally in line with our cheekbones, so circular motions will just drag the skin rather than work the muscles.)

PUFFINESS: If you wake up with puffy skin, place your fingertips in the centre of your face and work out towards your ears in a gentle patting motion. This will stimulate the lymphatic system, which lies just beneath the surface of the skin, and help to drain that excess fluid.

BAGGY EYES: Stroke the skin gently with your fingertips, working outwards from the inside of the eye socket. (If you do it the other way around, you'll make the bags worse.) Pinching along your brows will stop the upper eyelid sagging and lift the overall appearance of the brows.

NECK: Necks need as much TLC as your face. Treat yours to a regular massage, working upwards in smooth, sweeping stokes to get rid of any excess fluid.

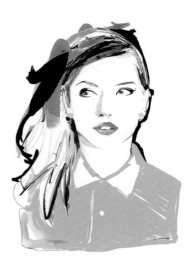

NICHOLA JOSS' FACIAL MASSAGE

I visit Nichola Joss' when I need an expert facial massage, but here she has given you a step-by-step guide to recreating this essential beauty treatment in your own home. With thanks to the Sanctuary Spa for the step-by-step illustrations.

#1

Pop 3–4 drops of facial oil into your palms and rub together to warm the oil a little.

#2

Close your eyes and hold your hands up to your face, taking a few deep breaths to enjoy the aroma of the oil.

#3

Gently press the palms of your hands to your face and move your hands outwards in smooth sweeping movements, working from the centre of the face outwards.

#4

Massage the oil into your skin for 1 minute using your fingertips then starting from the centre of the face, work outwards and upwards in small circular motions.

#5

To firm and tone the jawline, bend your index and middle fingers on both hands and place your chin between your knuckles. Glide along your jawline to under your ears in a sweeping motion. Repeat 6 times.

#6

To improve facial contours place the pads of your thumbs under your cheekbones with your palms facing outwards and gently push up. Work from the centre of the face outwards. Repeat 6 times.

#7

To improve fine lines and wrinkles across your brow area place your fingertips on the centre of your brow and with a firm pressure sweep upwards and outwards, moving towards the hairline and finishing at the temples. Repeat 6 times.

#8

Improve the firmness of the skin on the neck by gently using your palms to sweep the oil up the neck area.

#9

Then sweep your palms across your chest from left shoulder to right shoulder, sweeping across the décolletage with the palm of the hand. Repeat 3 times on both sides.

#10

Finally, sweep residual oil onto the back of your hands to improve the appearance of fine lines and wrinkles on hands.

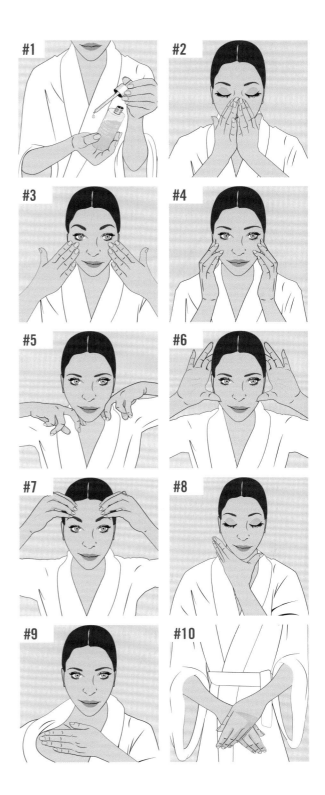

MILLIE'S MORNING CLEANSING ROUTINE

Everyone's routine is different. I love mine and it doesn't take that long. Here's what I do every morning:

#1

Rinse my face in warm water using a gentle foaming cleanser to remove any night oil or cream. (Hot water can make the capillaries come to the fore and irritate sensitive skin.)

#2

Rinse my face in cold water to close the pores and wake me up.

#3

Massage hydrating serum into my whole face to make it look plumped up and dewy.

#4

Clean my teeth while the serum is absorbed.

#5

Apply light day moisturiser with sun protection. (The type of moisturiser I use varies throughout the year and according to how my skin feels. I tend to use a gel in the summer and a richer cream in the winter. If I'm having a breakout, I'll go for one that's oil free.)

Make sure you cleanse every morning and night, devising your own routine to follow

MILLIE'S NIGHT-TIME CLEANSING ROUTINE

And this is what I do every night, no matter how late I get home:

#1

Remove my eye make-up using eye specific make-up remover and a cotton-wool ball.

#2

Massage my face all over with an oil-based cleanser and remove with a white muslin cloth (see page 83).

#3

I'm a big fan of double cleansing, so I will often repeat stage 2, particularly if I've been wearing a lot of make-up. Basically, if there are any traces of make-up on the cloth, then your face isn't clean.

#4

Massage two or three drops of oil into my face – I find this more hydrating than a night-time moisturiser. I try to find ones containing jojoba oil, which is really good for breakouts.

#5

Apply lip balm and hand cream.

Occasionally, I add in extra steps. For example, once or twice a week I like to use a mask in the evening. The type of mask I choose will depend on how my skin is feeling; quite often I'll use a hydrating one on my forehead and eye area and a deep-cleansing mud or clay one on my chin. Central heating and cold air dry out my skin, so I like to leave a hydrating mask on overnight once or twice a week during the winter and on flights.

COMMON SKIN PROBLEMS AND HOW TO TREAT OR BEAT THEM

Spots, dry patches, red patches, dull, lifeless-looking skin … Few of us are unaffected by these kind of skin issues and I've certainly had more than my fair share over the years. The upside of that is that I now have a long list of tried and tested problem-busting tips. Here are the best:

SPOTS

We all get the odd teenage spot or three. A few of us grew fringes to hide them, we all picked at them like crazy, and some people who had more than their fair share, like Miss Millie Mackintosh aged 13¾, cut up the membrane of a raw egg and plastered the bits across the offending blemishes. (Don't try it: it didn't work and looked ridiculous.) There's no getting away from it – spots are horrible. But there are things you can do to help.

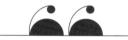

*Unfortunately, few of us
are unaffected by skin issues,
but you can learn ways to
help improve your skin*

94

HERE ARE MY TOP TEN DOS AND DON'TS FOR BREAKOUTS:

#1 DON'T use strong toning products designed to strip oil out of the skin. It may sound like a good idea to use them, because it's excess oil that is causing the problem, but in fact by stripping the oil out, you are just dehydrating your skin and your body will produce more to compensate.

#2 DO keep your skin as clean as possible. Cleanse night and morning with a foaming cleanser (look for one that's gentle and mildly anti-bacterial).

#3 DON'T squeeze. You may think you're getting the bacteria out, but you are more likely to spread the infection by pushing it further into the spot.

#4 DON'T overload your skin with products. Too many different products can upset your skin, leading to more breakouts.

#5 DO let your skin breath.

#6 DON'T ignore your diet. What you eat affects your skin – mine reacts badly to too much sugar.

#7 DO drink lots of water and seek out foods rich in vitamin C (such as dark leafy greens and berries) and zinc (such as meat, shellfish and cheese).

#8 DON'T underestimate the power of a good night's sleep – skin repairs itself while we sleep. I try to get to bed by 10 p.m. at the latest whenever I am in for the evening.

#9 DO keep stress to a minimum. It's hard to avoid, but meditation, slow yoga and breathing exercises (see pages 274–279) will keep you calm.

#10 DO keep a tray of toner ice cubes in your freezer. The combination of ice and toner really helps to dry out a spot, so when a horror strikes, simply remove one from the ice-cube tray and hold over the offending pimple.

HERE ARE MY TOP TEN DOS AND DON'TS FOR DRY SKIN:

#1 DON'T use steam rooms and avoid spending too long in the shower or bath. The problem is that hot water strips your body of its natural oil barrier and you need that barrier to help trap moisture and keep your skin smooth and moist. So dial down the temperature and don't linger too long. Skin-care experts recommend short, warm showers or baths that last no longer than 5–10 minutes.

#2 DO use rich cream or oil cleansers.

#3 DON'T go out in the sun without a broad-spectrum SPF 30 sunscreen. Ever. Sun damage is one of the main causes of rough, dry skin and wrinkles.

#4 DO exfoliate but always use a gentle product designed specifically for dry skin.

#5 DON'T scrub too hard.

#6 DO try using a serum containing hyaluronic acid. This will target the dryness from beneath the skin's surface and plump out fine lines.

#7 DON'T ignore your diet. Up your intake of naturally oil-rich foods such as avocados and fatty fish like salmon, and snack on nuts, seeds and antioxidant-rich berries.

#8 DO try to drink 2 litres of water every day.

#9 DON'T overheat your house. Central heating removes moisture from the air, which can leave dry skin even more parched. Consider using a humidifier in your bedroom too. Indoor humidity should be about 50 per cent – you can keep track of moisture levels easily with an inexpensive device called a hygrometer.

#10 DO try adding a drop of facial oil to your moisturiser or switch to using oil at night.

how to make a shocker
go away sharpish

It's happened to all of us: you wake up on the morning of an important event and find that you've grown a whopper overnight. When this happens, DO NOT SQUEEZE (unless the white head literally looks as if it's going to burst through your skin); try one of these tricks instead:

★ Cover the head of the spot with a tissue and tap gently until the pus comes out naturally.

★ Dab on a mixture of white wine vinegar and tea tree oil. The vinegar will dry the spot out and the tea tree oil acts as a disinfectant.

★ Break out the toner ice cubes (see page 95).

★ Mix a dollop of plain yoghurt with a couple of crushed aspirin and some manuka honey, apply to the offending pimple and leave for 15 minutes. Wash clean.

DULL SKIN

Dull skin is probably a sign that you are tired and stressed. But don't panic – here are four simple revitalising rules:

DO exfoliate. Dead skin cells build up over time if you don't remove them. Go and read the section on exfoliators for more on this (see page 85)!

DON'T skimp on your sleep.

DO use a brightening serum or moisturiser with ingredients specifically designed to target dark spots and dullness.

DON'T forget the power of make-up. Apply a primer with tiny shimmer particles (we're not talking face glitter – these are so small you can't even see them) under your base. Finish off with a powder or cream highlighter (see page 126 for more on this).

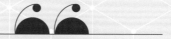

Learn to identify the symptoms of your skin (dull, dry or sensitive) and always treat it appropriately

SENSITIVE SKIN

Sensitive skin needs lots of TLC and there are several different conditions that might affect it, from rosacea to eczema. For most people, treatment will involve both self-help measures (see below) and medication. I would always recommend seeing a dermatologist, particularly if the specialist products you've tried haven't worked.

DON'T use too many different products. I recently suffered from dermatitis, which is a skin condition that looks similar to eczema, around my nose and chin. It was caused by a combination of too many products, cold weather and central heating.

DO think about your washing detergents. Switching to washing liquid designed for baby's skin helped clear up my dermatitis.

DON'T forget to test. If you haven't used a product before, do a patch test on the inside of your wrist and see how your skin reacts.

DO try moisturising with pure jojoba oil. This was a tip from my facialist, Nataliya Robinson. Lots of skin conditions are caused by fungal infections and jojoba oil is not only nourishing but has anti-fungal properties too.

DON'T ignore your diet. It's worth cutting out common triggers like alcohol, caffeine and dairy to see whether things improve.

DO seek professional advice from your GP or a dermatologist. There are several medical treatments available, ranging from topical creams and gels to oral antibiotics and laser and IPL (intense pulsed light) therapy, both of which involve shrinking visible blood vessels by subjecting them to beams of light.

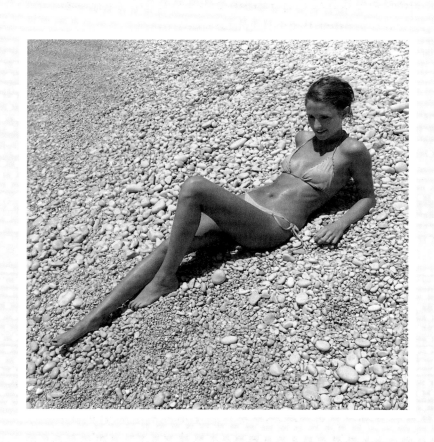

BODY

Just like the skin on your face, the skin on your body needs looking after. Body skin care is pretty straightforward – it's really just a question of exfoliating and moisturising.

EXFOLIATING

Exfoliating is quick, easy and, done regularly, will keep your skin looking bright and feeling smooth. What's not to love?

BODY BRUSHING

I like to use a body brush two or three times a week, because not only does it get rid of dead skin cells, it also increases circulation, helps to combat cellulite and improves the overall texture of the skin. Brush towards your heart in a firm, sweeping motion before you get in the shower. (The shower will wash away both the skin cells and the toxins released by all that brushing.)

BODY SCRUBS

These are really nourishing for the skin and are brilliant at removing the remnants of a fake tan. I tend to use a scrub once or twice a week. Apply before you shower using a hand mitt or a Clarisonic body brush for really deep penetration, and rub in large, circular motions. Pay particular attention to dry areas such as ankles, knees and elbows. Body scrubs tend to be either salt or sugar based; sugar is gentle enough for sensitive skin, whereas salt is perfect for stubborn areas such as heels and elbows.

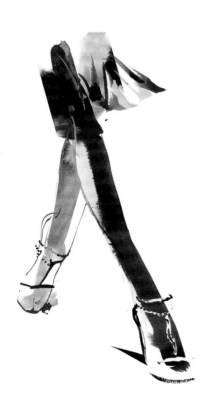

MOISTURISING

I moisturise all over, every day. I use my face moisturiser for my neck and décolletage, where the skin is thinner, and then a body oil or moisturiser everywhere else. (Moisturiser is absorbed more quickly than oil so is better if you're in a hurry.) In the winter, I use a more intensive cream on areas prone to dryness, such as my shins.

HOLIDAY SKIN CARE

Just because you are going away, it doesn't mean that you have to change your beauty regime. I have a big beauty bag and just decant all my daily products into mini bottles so I can take them with me. However, if you're going to a different climate, you will want to adjust your products accordingly. For example, if you are heading off somewhere hot, then you will need some super-hydrating moisturiser with added sun protection. Avoid anything exfoliating because it will make you skin more susceptible to burning. If you are going somewhere cold, you will then need a nourishing and protective moisturiser.

HOME PAMPERING

There's nothing quite like a spot of pampering to make a girl feel good – and while spa days are fabulous, you can do a pretty good DIY one too. This is my tried and tested, top-secret, at-home treat:

★ Run a warm bath full of lovely essential oils, surrounded by candles (if you have dry skin, don't sit for too long).

★ Meanwhile, give my body a good buff with an indulgent exfoliator (see page 101).

★ Get in the bath, washing off the exfoliator. Sit for ages and relax while the pores open up – hard work but someone's got to do it!

★ Apply a nourishing hair mask (see page 110).

★ Give my face a really good wash and massage (see page 83 and 90) to remove the day's make-up and drain the toxins.

★ Exfoliate. I use the amazing REN Glycolactic Skin Renewal Peel Mask, which contains loads of fruit acids to gently dissolve dead skin cells.

★ Remove any remaining gunk with a clean muslin cloth or flannel.

★ Apply a face mask, such as Bliss's Triple Oxygen Instant Energising Mask.

★ Get out of the bath, wrap up in a warm, fluffy towel.

★ Moisturise my body all over with body oil.

★ Apply serum to my face, followed by a nourishing night oil.

★ Meditate (see page 278).

★ Sleep for 10 hours. Lovely!

FAKE TAN

I like to maintain a light, golden glow all year round because having a tan makes me feel happy. I think I caught the brown bug from my grannies, one of whom still uses a moisturiser with a tanning ingredient every day. (She puts it on my grandfather too!)

Here are my top tips for a natural-looking home tan:

SHAVE: It's best to do this the day before you plan to tan. If you apply it to freshly shaved legs, it will sink into the hair follicles, leaving them covered with dark brown dots.

EXFOLIATE: The tanning product will otherwise stick to any dry patches, leaving you with dark blotches, so you must be thorough. I use an exfoliating mask with fruit acids for my face, but you could use a scrub. If so, apply it with your fingers and rub in a circular motion, paying particular attention to your chin and around your nose. Body scrubs are best applied to dry skin, then rinsed off in the shower.

MOISTURISE: Rub a tiny drop of moisturiser to your ankles, knees, knuckles, wrists, elbows and armpits. This will act as barrier so the tan won't sink too deeply into these areas.

DO A PATCH TEST: If you haven't used a product before, try a small amount somewhere that won't be seen before covering your entire body with it. If unsure, choose an instant tan that you can wash off.

APPLY EVENLY: You might like to use a tanning mitt to help smooth away any lines.

BE PATIENT: Some tans take a couple of hours to develop, so wait before adding more. You might want to build the tan up over a couple of days.

FESTIVAL SKIN CARE

Space is tight and access to bathrooms – or even water – severely limited, so festivals call for an SOS kit. This is mine:

MAKE-UP WIPES: These are too harsh for everyday use, but perfect for dry cleansing.

GEL-FILLED EYE MASK: Blocks out the light and combats baggy eyes.

DRY SHAMPOO: Choose a clear one that won't leave a powdery residue.

WATER MIST: Just the thing for reviving a tired face.

HAND SANITISER: You know why.

SUNGLASSES AND HATS: To hide any disasters.

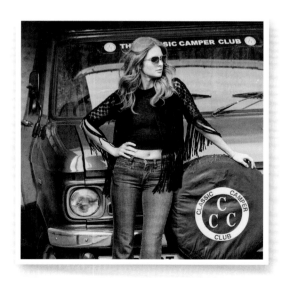

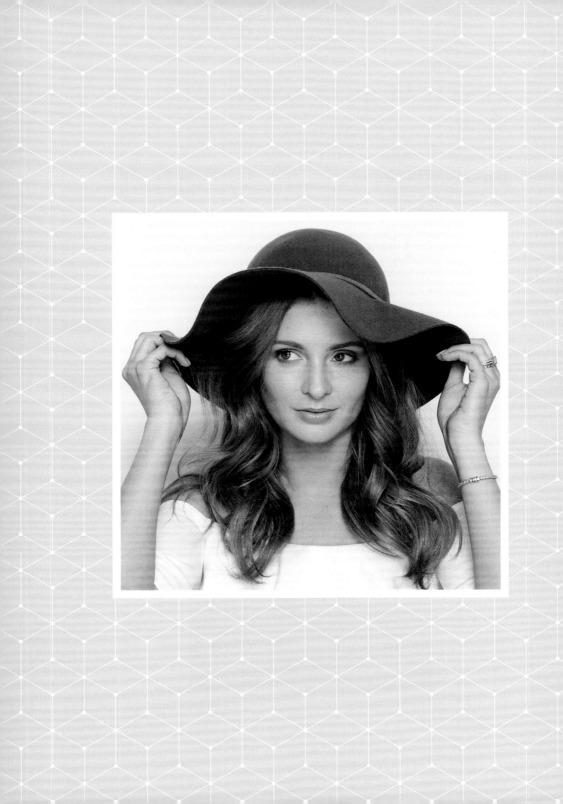

HAIR

How you look after your hair will depend on its type and style – mine is mid-length and frizzy. I use a sulphate- and paraben-free shampoo and conditioner and I try not to wash it every day because it can strip out the natural oils and make it dry. After shoots when I've had loads of product in it, I use a clarifying shampoo to give it a deep clean.

Here are some basic dos and don'ts:

DO protect your hair with a heat-protection product when you're using styling tools or are out in the sun.

DON'T leave chlorine or sea salt on your hair after swimming. As great as sea-salt dried beachy waves look, salt water really does dry out your hair.

DO use a 30-minute hair mask once a week. I like to leave one in overnight sometimes too, and if you use one while you're sunbathing, it acts like a heat treatment. (See pages 110–112 for recipes for my homemade hair masks.)

DON'T put lemon juice on your hair. Ever. It may be a natural product, but it works just like bleach.

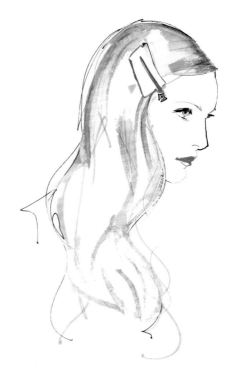

CUTTING

There are two key rules when it comes to finding the style for you:

 # LOOK AT YOUR FACE AND HAIR: It's all very well finding a great hair cut in a magazine or deciding that you want a sleek bob because it's in fashion, but you need to be sure that the shape will suit your hair type and your face. I found this out the hard way just after I got married when I decided I wanted a fringe. It was a frizzy disaster and I couldn't grow it out fast enough.

 # FIND YOURSELF A HAIRDRESSER YOU CAN TRUST: This means someone honest enough to tell you that the sleek bob is not a good idea. I go for a trim every eight weeks to get rid of split ends and I find that it takes a couple of weeks to settle after a cut, so I time my trips to the salon accordingly.

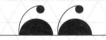

*Looking after your hair
is just as important as
looking after your skin*

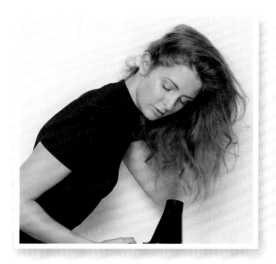
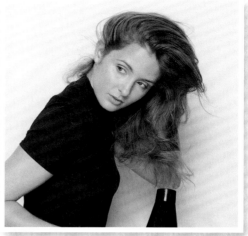

HOW TO ADD VOLUME TO FINE HAIR

\# Use volumising shampoos and conditioners.

\# Use a mousse or root spray on damp hair before styling.

\# Rough-dry your hair with your head upside down.

\# Add texture to your hair by drying it with a hair dryer and running your fingers through it rather than using a brush, which can make it too flat.

\# Use a texturising spray to give it enough body to hold curls or waves.

\# Try heated rollers.

\# Experiment with clip-in extensions. These are a great way of adding more volume and length for a special occasion and, unlike permanent extensions, they are maintenance free and don't weaken your hair.

HOW TO TAME FRIZZY HAIR

Use a frizz-beating shampoo and conditioner.

After washing, towel-dry your hair and add a small amount
of serum from roots to ends.

Smooth out with a hair dryer and brush, then go over your hair
in sections with straighteners.

Try a Brazilian blow dry (this usually contains keratin) at your hair
salon. But bear in mind that this only works on thick hair and some
treatments can be damaging, so do some research first.

SPECIAL TREATMENTS

Constant heating, styling and colouring is bad for our hair, so if you
want to keep your locks looking luscious, it's worth treating them to
a mask from time to time. Here are three great hair masks that you
can make with ingredients you probably already have in your kitchen.

HOT OIL

This is a really deep treatment for dry, damaged hair and dry scalps.
Warming the oil means that it penetrates the hair follicles. Use once
or twice a month.

How to make

The type of oil you use depends on your hair type. For example, sweet
almond, argan or extra-virgin coconut oil are all good for normal hair;
castor oil is perfect for oily hair; and dry or coarse hair is best treated
with jojoba or avocado oil. You can also use a mixture – one of my
favourites is coconut and almond. The amount you use also varies

according to hair type and length but a little goes a long way. Somewhere between a teaspoon and a tablespoon should be enough.

How to apply
Wet your hair so that it is damp rather than soaking and remove any styling products that may stop the mask working so well.

Warm the oil in small bowl placed in a larger bowl of boiling water – 10 minutes should do it. You want it hot enough to penetrate, but not so hot that it burns your scalp.

Massage the oil into your hair and scalp, working from the roots to the ends. Wrap your head in a plastic shower cap or cling film and cover with a towel. (Warm the towel first in the airing cupboard or with a hair dryer.)

Relax for 20–30 minutes.

Wash with shampoo. You will need to do this at least twice, but trust me – the results are worth it.

EGG YOLK PROTEIN
This mask is packed with protein, vitamins and super-nurturing fatty acids, all of which will make your hair softer, shinier and healthier. An abundance of vitamins A, D and E will prevent any hair loss and promote new growth, as well as keeping split ends at bay. Olive oil also strengthens and softens, making this mask particularly good for treating dry or damaged hair. And as if all that weren't enough, it also exfoliates your tresses, intensifies the colour and maintains texture. Do this once a month.

How to make
Mix 2 egg yolks with 2 tablespoons of olive oil, then dilute the mixture with half a cup of water. (Separate the egg by cracking it and passing

the yolk from shell half to shell half, letting the white fall into a bowl. Alternatively, simply crack the egg and pour it into your hand, allowing the white to run through your fingers.)

How to apply
Wet your hair so that it's damp rather than soaking, then slowly massage the mask into your scalp, working from the roots to the ends.

Let it set for 15–20 minutes, but without covering your hair – you don't want the egg to cook!

Wash out thoroughly using shampoo and conditioner.

AVOCADO AND HONEY

This is an excellent moisturising and strengthening treatment for dry and brittle hair. Avocados are loaded with nutritious oils, while honey is naturally high in vitamins and minerals and helps your hair to retain water and moisture. Olive oil is both moisturising and protecting. If your hair is badly damaged, I suggest doing this once a week until you see an improvement, then once a month after that.

How to make
Mash a large, ripe avocado with a fork until you have a smooth purée, then gradually stir in a tablespoon of raw honey and a tablespoon of oil (olive, argan, coconut – whatever you have to hand).

How to apply
Wet your hair with warm water and massage the mixture evenly, working from the roots downwards, paying attention to the ends.

Cover with a shower cap, if you have one, or cling film.

Grab a book and a cup of tea and relax for 35–45 minutes.

Wash well with shampoo.

TO DYE FOR

What is it about at-home hair colour that makes it universally irresistible to teenage girls? No, peroxide blonde won't work if you're a dark brunette, and yes, it's actually pretty easy to turn your hair orange or blue or purple.

I am speaking from experience. When I was about 13, I was at a friend's house for the weekend and she had a packet of DIY hair dye. It was called Ash Blonde. Well, the result for yours truly was a fluorescent yellow, brittle, frizzy mess and the only remedy was a long and expensive programme of more dyes and treatments. First I had it dyed brown, but the bleach in the Ash Blonde caused it to fade really quickly, so I then had to keep having a blend of highlights and lowlights put in until the original dye grew out. I learned my lesson.

My hair has been my natural colour for a few years now and it's in really great condition, so I have no intention of dyeing it. If I did, though, I would definitely have it done professionally. Anyone thinking about dyeing their hair should consider popping into a wig shop to try out different colours. It is also important to do a patch test on a piece of hair at the back of your neck to see how your hair will react to the colour. And before you do it, be aware that dyed hair is high maintenance. Not only will you be making regular trips to the salon to keep your roots topped up, you will also have to invest time, money and energy in caring for your hair with nourishing products.

MILLIE'S SIGNATURE HAIRSTYLES

A change of hairstyle can transform a look. And it's free too!
Here are four of my favourites.

MILLIE'S LOVELY LOOSE CURLS

This is my everyday style. I like to do it a while, preferably a few hours, before I go out to give it time to drop a bit; indeed it often looks better the next day, revived with some dry shampoo and a bit of light curling with tongs.

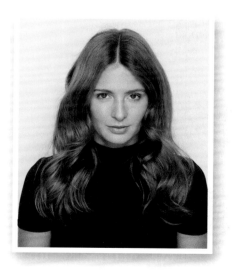

#1

Wash and roughly dry your hair, then tip your head upside down and blow dry from the roots to give it the maximum volume.

#2

Part down the centre and tong on both sides, working from the back of your head towards your face.

#3

Loosen through with your fingers.

#1

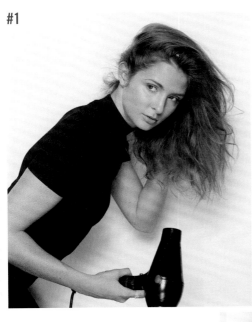

#2

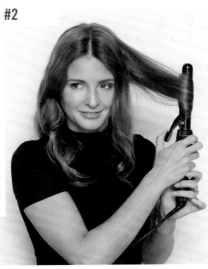

#3

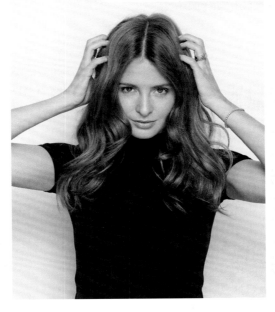

MILLIE'S BRILLIANT BRAIDS

This is my go-to hairstyle for festivals and weddings.

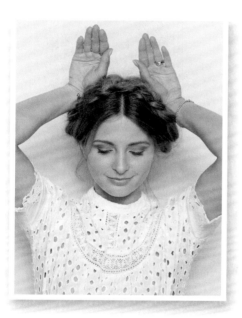

#1

Part your hair and braid into two plaits, starting at the bottom of your ears.

#2

Loosen each braid with your fingers.

#3

Cross each plait over on top of your head, fold and pin in place.

#1

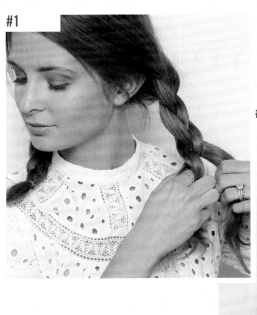

#2

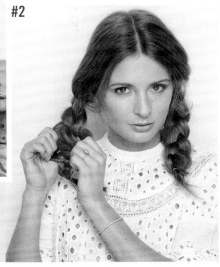

#3

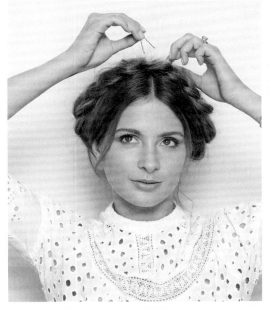

MILLIE'S MARVELLOUS MESSY BUN

Messy buns are really versatile – great during the day worn with jeans, T-shirt and heels, and brilliant for dressing down a posh frock.

#1

Tip your head upside down and create a ponytail on top of your head.

#2

Twist the ponytail round and pin.

#3

Pull the bun apart with your fingers to create a loose, messy bun.

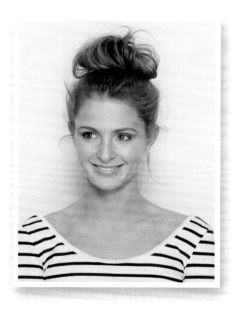

#1

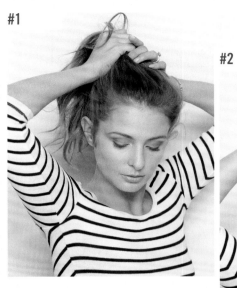

#2

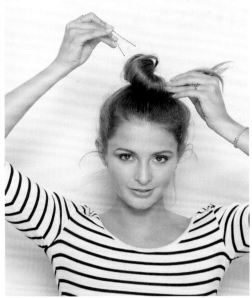

#3

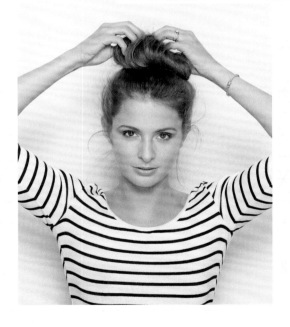

MILLIE'S PROPER PONYTAIL

A ponytail will sharpen up an evening look. I like to wear one with a dress or suit, finished off with my signature smoky eye or red lip (see pages 142 and 138).

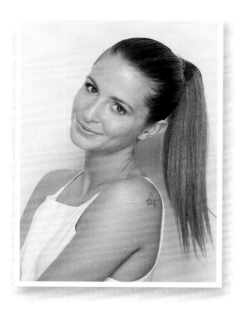

#1

Comb your hair back off your face and spray it with hair spray to give a clean, sharp finish.

#2

Pull your hair back into a ponytail and secure with a band.

#3

I sometimes like to wrap a hair extension weft round the top of the ponytail for extra volume and thickness, which you can then secure to the ponytail with pins.

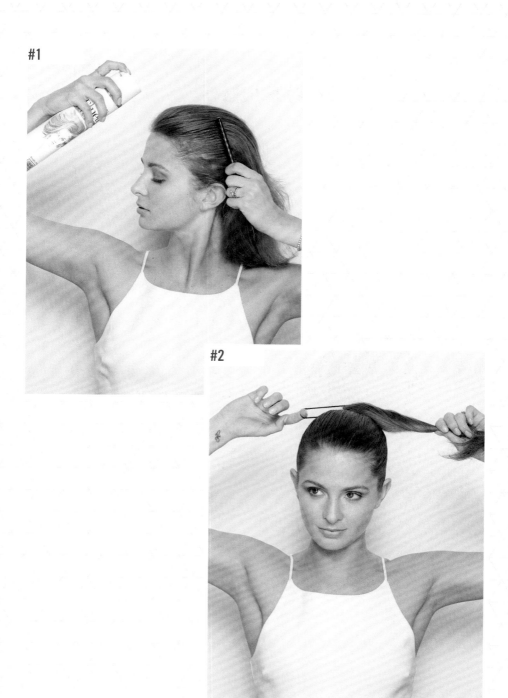

#1

#2

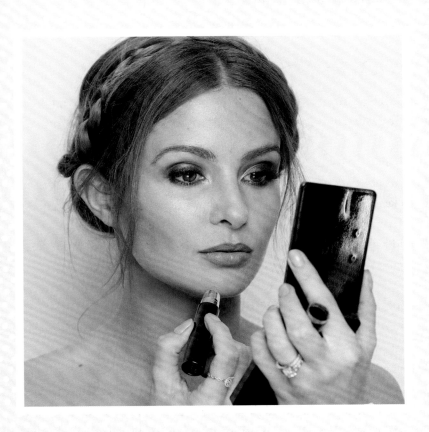

MAKE-UP

Make-up can enhance, conceal and transform our faces. This section is all about showing you how.

MAKE-UP BAG ESSENTIALS

With so many products, it is easy (and fun) to get carried away, but here are the items I think every girl's make-up bag should contain.

PRIMER

This goes under your foundation or tinted moisturiser and its job is to keep your make-up in place all day. There are primers to regulate oil, primers with sun protection, primers to hydrate and primers to add a glow – just choose the one that best suits your skin type (see page 78). Apply it with your fingers.

FOUNDATION/TINTED MOISTURISER

These days, I prefer tinted moisturisers for my everyday look because they just even out skin tone without looking too perfect. I always use one with added sun protection. Whichever you go for, it's vital to get the colour right. I always test it on my forehead, cheek, neck and chin. Find some natural light too – if that's difficult in the shop, ask to take some away in a sample pot. Remember that your skin changes colour through the year, so your base needs to change too. Apply with your fingers or a foundation buffing brush (see page 127).

CONCEALER

Concealer is available in lots of different consistencies, but I like to use a creamy one under my eyes and a thicker one to hide any blemishes. Some come with an applicator, but I find tapping the cream lightly with my fingertips works best under my eyes. I use a small brush for blemishes. You need to buy two shades – one with slightly reflective qualities for under your eyes (this will draw attention away from the bags) and a darker, non-reflective one for covering blemishes.

BRONZER

I'm a big fan of bronzers because they really warm up your face. The secret of success is to think about how the sun hits your face and apply your bronzer in the same places – i.e. your forehead, nose and cheekbones. Apply with a big brush.

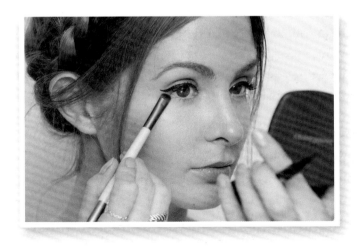

BLUSHER

Blusher adds colour to your cheeks. When you're choosing the colour, think about what colour your face goes when it's tanned. Apply with a brush from the apple of your cheek out towards the cheekbone. I use a powder blusher but you can get creams. If you do choose a cream, then you need to use a cream bronzer too, because you can't put cream over powder.

TINTED EYEBROW GEL

There are lots of products on the market, from pencils to shadows. I like gel because it fills out your eyebrows and keeps them in place.

EYE SHADOW AND TONING EYE PENCIL

I have green eyes, so I go for warm shades of brown, orange and aubergine. Bronze shades are good for bringing out blue eyes, while dark charcoal greys are lovely with brown eyes.

EYELINER

Buy one in a creamy, nude shade for using along your waterline (the line of your lower lid that sits between the lashes and the eye itself). This makes your eyes look bigger and more awake. (A bit of highlighting powder in the inner corners will do this too.) A black kohl eyeliner is also essential for adding some drama.

MASCARA

I love mascara and usually wear one with a purple tint to bring out the green accents in my eyes. Volumising ones with a thick brush, like Charlotte Tilbury's Full Fat Lashes mascara, are great for accentuating your eyes. I like to use a bit of mascara even if I'm wearing false lashes – it helps them blend in with my own eyelashes.

FALSE EYELASHES

I'm a big fan of false eyelashes and there are eight different styles in my line. If your want a subtle look, choose lashes that match your own and always buy ones made with natural hair. All lashes come as a standard length, so you will need to trim them to the right size – just peel off the packet, hold them against your eye and cut with nail scissors. You can use individual lashes to fill out your own or add impact at the corners.

LIPSTICK, LIP GLOSS AND LIP PENCILS

Lip pencils should always be as close in colour to your lipstick as possible. Drawing a subtle line just outside the natural lip line will make your lips appear fuller. Filling in your lips with lip pencil before you apply lipstick will make it last longer, while using a lip pencil followed by lip gloss creates a natural nude lip (see pages 140–141).

HIGHLIGHTING POWDER

Brush over the inner corners of your eye to open them up and over your brow bone to accentuate your eyebrows. I also like to dust a bit down the centre of my nose, on the tops of my cheekbones and on my Cupid's bow.

TRANSLUCENT POWDER

This is good for dusting over your T-zone (see page 78) to prevent shine. It's also brilliant for dusting under your eyes to protect your face when you're creating a smoky eye (see pages 142–143).

BRUSHES

Different brushes do different things, so you need a selection. You can build your collection over time; you don't need to buy all of these at once! These are the ones that I use:

FOUNDATION BRUSHES AND SPONGES: I like to put tinted moisturiser on with my fingers, but I use both brushes and sponges for thicker foundations. Flat-headed brushes buff make-up into the skin and give really even coverage (blend afterwards with your fingers for a super-smooth finish). Foundation sponges, which you use slightly damp, work in the same way.

LARGE POWDER BRUSHES: These are good for applying both translucent powder and bronzer because they disperse the powder evenly over a large area of skin. You need to have two separate brushes – one for powder and one for bronzer.

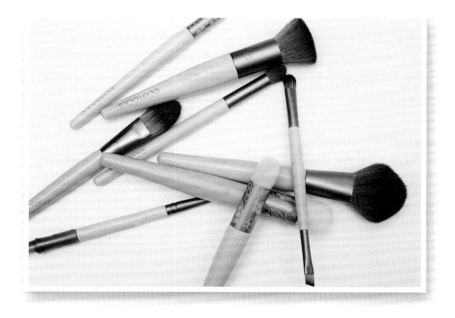

CONTOUR BRUSHES: These are angled to make it easier to apply bronzer or highlighter under the cheekbone.

BLUSHER BRUSHES: Designed to be used just on your cheek rather than your whole face, these are slightly smaller than contour and powder brushes.

SMALL POWDER BRUSHES: These are ideal for getting in round your nose and chin and for when you just want to do a quick touch-up.

EYEBROW BRUSHES: A must-have for keeping your brows in order.

EYE-SHADOW APPLICATOR BRUSHES: You need two large ones for applying eye shadow (one for dark shades, one for light), plus a small one for blending underneath the eye.

EYELINER BRUSHES: You should have one of these even if you use an eyeliner pen because they're great for creating the Feline Flick powder-tracing line (see page 136).

EYE-SHADOW BLENDING BRUSHES: These are rounded brushes which you use after you've applied the shadow to create a smooth finish. (You can't use the applicator brush because it will be full of powder.)

FAN BRUSHES: Shaped like a fan, these are designed to flick specks of stray make-up away from under your eyes.

OTHER ITEMS

Your beauty kit should also contain:

 # EYELASH CURLERS – for the best effect, heat the curler for 10 seconds before using. Check it's not too hot before you use it and remember – curl your lashes before you apply mascara.

 # TWEEZERS – for keeping your eyebrows in shape (see page 130 for more on eyebrow care) and for applying false eyelashes.

 # MAGNIFYING MIRROR

 # NAIL POLISH

 # ORANGE STICKS – a manicure tool for cleaning fingernails and pushing back cuticles.

 # CUTICLE OIL – to keep cuticles soft and hydrated.

 # HAND CREAM

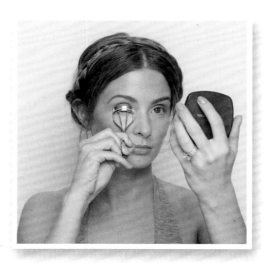

EYEBROWS

Eyebrows frame your eyes and face. Over the years, I have experienced a fair few mishaps due to over-plucking my brows: they've been too thin, too far apart or too short at the ends – none of which are good looks, believe me. So, to help you avoid making similar mistakes, I asked make-up artist Justine Jenkins for her top 5 tips.

#1

Always follow your natural brow shape and do not over-pluck. This is my rule of thumb: place a pencil along the outside of your nostril straight up to your brow and remove any hairs growing from the area between the edge of the pencil and the centre of your face. Then move the end of the pencil towards the outer corner of your eye and remove any hairs outside the pencil line. If you're still unsure which hairs to remove, draw over them with a flesh-coloured pencil so that you can check the shape before removing.

#2

Never pluck the top of your brows. You want to create a good arched shape, so always pluck from underneath.

#3

Remember, eyebrows are sisters not twins – they don't have to be perfect and match each other exactly.

#4

Invest in an eyebrow comb to keep stray hairs in order.

#5

Disinfect your tweezers – they carry traces of dirt and make-up that can cause breakouts.

NAILS

How your nails look is just as important as how you do your face and what you're wearing. There's no point in having flawless make-up and an amazing outfit if your nails are scuzzy and bitten, girls. It's all about appearing groomed at all times, and a flawless manicure is an easy way to give the impression that you are 100 per cent fabulous. Here are some top tips for nail perfection:

#1

Soak your hands for 5 minutes in warm, soapy water. Gently push back the cuticles using an orange stick. Be careful not to cut your cuticles.

#2

Apply a base coat onto dry nails.

#3

Apply two thin coats of polish, followed by a fast-drying top coat.

#4

Use hand cream daily.

#5

Use nourishing cuticle oil daily. Keep it by your bed so you don't forget.

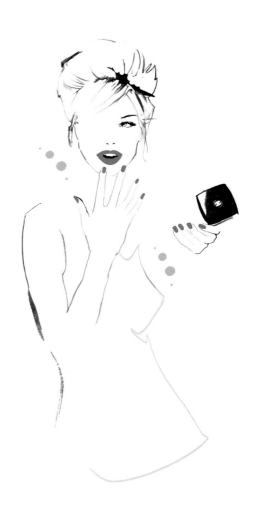

MILLIE'S SIGNATURE LOOKS

MILLIE'S EVERYDAY FACE

I wore such heavy make-up in my teens that my face was basically a mask. These days, I've come to realise that a natural look is much more flattering, so while I love to go all out at parties, for every day I have mastered a way of enhancing my features and improving the look of my skin while letting my own, natural face come through. It takes me five minutes and I can virtually do it in my sleep! Here's a step-by-step guide:

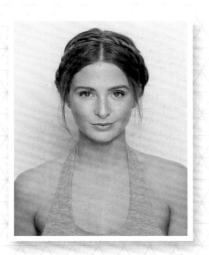

#1 PRIMER

Apply an illuminating primer to your whole face for a light, subtle glow.

#2 TINTED MOISTURISER

Apply tinted moisturiser with sun protection to your whole face.

#3 CONCEALER

Concealer – cream for under the eyes; stick concealer for blemishes.

#4 TRANSLUCENT POWDER

Brush translucent powder along the T-zone (see page 78) and over any blemishes to set the make-up.

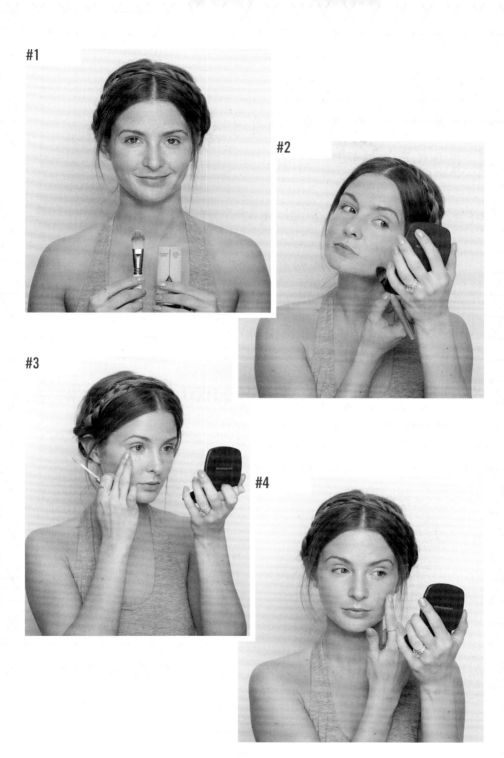

#5

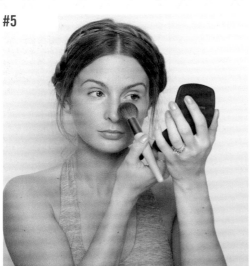

#6

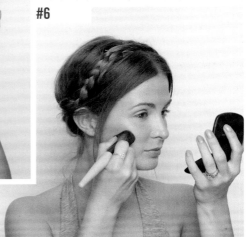

#7

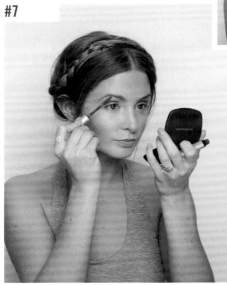

#8

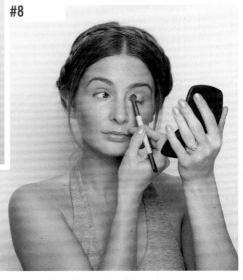

#5 BRONZER

Brush bronzer across your forehead, temples, cheekbones and underneath the jaw so that your neck colour matches your face.

#6 BLUSHER

Brush blusher on the apples of your cheeks – a peachy pink suits my skin tone.

#7 TINTED EYEBROW GEL

Apply tinted eyebrow gel to fill out your brows and keep them tidy.

#8 BRONZER

Brush bronzer, using a blending brush, along the socket lines of your eyes. This gives a more natural look than eye shadow.

#9 EYELINER

Draw inside the bottom waterline using a creamy, skin-tone eyeliner. This will make the eye appear more open.

#10 MASCARA

Apply mascara.

#11 GLOSS

Apply lip gloss.

#9

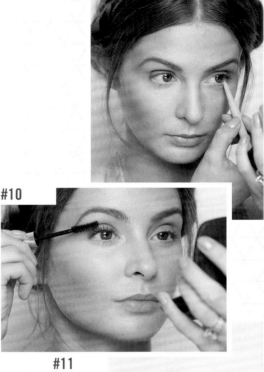

#10

#11

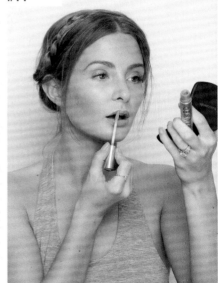

MILLIE'S FELINE FLICK

A black flick draws out the eye and makes lashes appear fuller. This a great way to pep up your face for an evening out after work.

#1
Apply the Everyday Face (see pages 132–135).

#2
Stretch out your eyelid and draw along the top lid using a liquid eyeliner. Work from the inner corner outwards, going as close to your lashes as possible, and stop where your lashes finish.

#3
It's really important to get the angle of the flick right – draw it wrong and you'll find that you just make yourself look tired. This is my fail-safe tip for success: dip a small eyeliner brush into translucent powder, line it up with your lower lash line and trace out along it, continuing at the same angle, until you reach the point where you upper lashes finish.

#4
Draw over the outer end of your powder line with liquid liner. You can tidy up any smudges with a cotton bud soaked in eye make-up remover.

#5
When your flick is perfect (and you can make it as subtle or as heavy as you like), remove the powder with a clean fan brush or dry cotton bud.

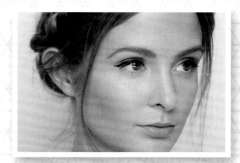

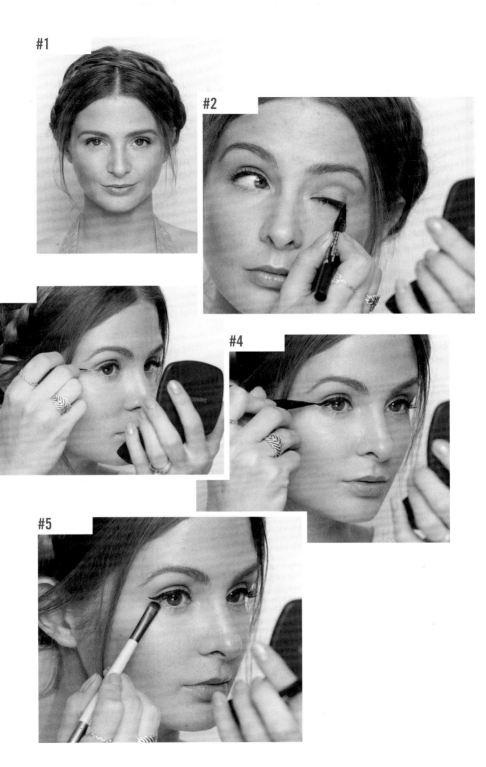

MILLIE'S RED LIP

Nothing dresses your face up quite like red lips. I like to pair them with my Everyday Face (see pages 132–135) for serious business meetings and with a Feline Flick or Smoky Eye (see pages 136 and 142) for sophisticated evening glamour. And in summer you can't beat a tanned face worn with nothing but a bright red, matt lip. Shades of lipstick range from nude pinks to vampy plums, and what you choose is up to you. Orange tones suit my skin colour.

#1

Pat your lips with your fingertips to make sure there's no product on them. If necessary, do a lip scrub. Using a lip pencil as close to your lipstick colour as possible, draw round the outside of the lip, starting from the Cupid's bow. Drawing the line very slightly outside the natural lip line will make your lips appear fuller.

#2

Colour your lips in roughly with the pencil. This will help your lipstick last longer.

#3

If you make a mistake, you can clean up with a cotton bud dipped in cleanser.

#4

Apply lipstick, again working outwards from your Cupid's bow.

#5

Blot with tissue. Stick your finger in your mouth and then pull it out – this stops any lipstick from getting on your teeth.

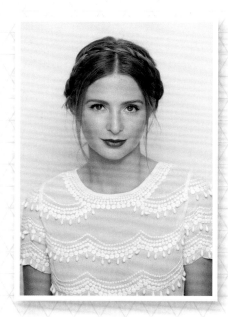

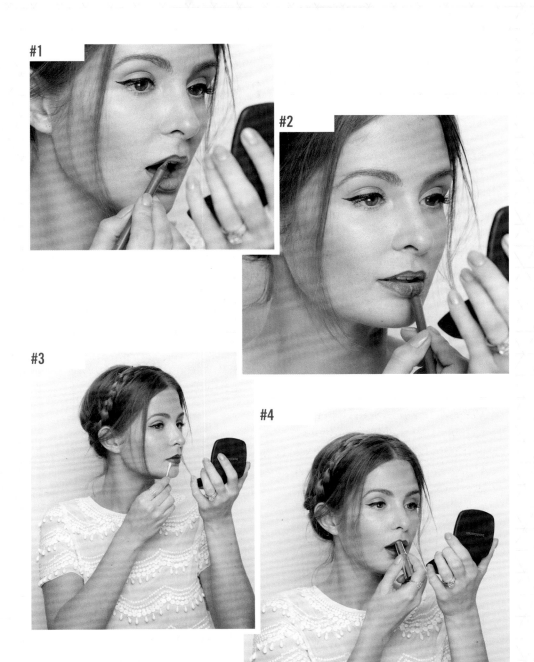

#1

#2

#3

#4

MILLIE'S NUDE LIP

Nude lips are the new classic. They are universally flattering and can brighten and bring together the most dressed down of looks. If going out, I like to pair nude lips with a dramatic smoky eye (see page 142).

#1

Pat your lips with your fingertips to make sure there's no product on them. If necessary, do a lip scrub. Using a lip pencil as close to your lip colour as possible, draw round the outside of the lip, starting from the Cupid's bow.

#2

Apply a neutral or nude lipstick, again working outwards from your Cupid's bow.

#3

Press your lips together and wipe away any excess lipstick, or mistakes.

Millie's festival face

Doing your face at a festival isn't easy, so I like to have a fake tan and some eyelash extensions before I go, then all I need to do is add a bit of glitter and a nude lip. Gel glitter is easy to use and is great on eyes and cheekbones.

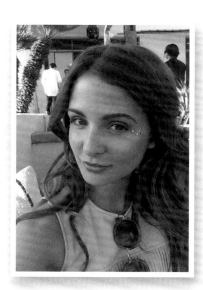

#1

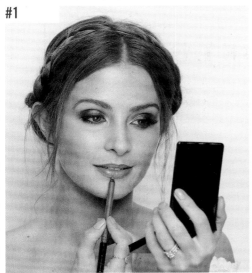

#2

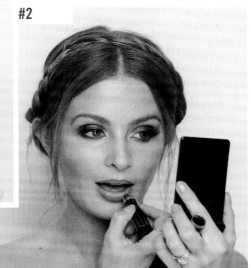

#3

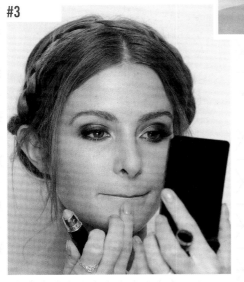

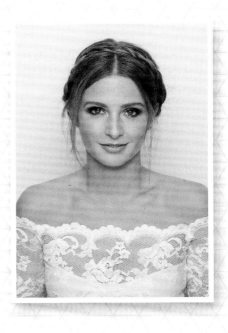

MILLIE'S SMOKY EYE

This is my go-to party look:

#1

Start with a bare face if possible,
particularly if you are less
experienced, so that if you end up
with eye shadow all over your face
you can just wash it off. However,
if you are already wearing your
Everyday Face (see pages 132–135),
just brush some translucent powder
under your eyes and dust off
afterwards. (If you do end up with
specks of powder on your face,
clean off with a dry cotton bud
and touch up with concealer.)

#2

Choose a base colour. I have green
eyes so I always go for dark bronzy
browns. (See page 125 for a note on
colours.) Using a large eye-shadow
brush, apply a wash of colour over
your eyelid, taking it right into
the socket line.

#3

Using a small blending brush or
pencil, draw the same colour under
the lower lash line and blend. You
want the colour to be slightly
darker at the edges.

#4

Draw along the top lash line with
a thick eyeliner pencil in a slightly
darker shade of your base colour.
Blend with your fingers.

#5

Trace along the inside of the lower
eye line with an eyeliner pencil.

#6

Add false lashes to accentuate the
corner of your eye. (Corner lashes
are shorter, so you will need to trim
the falsies with nail scissors.) Apply
the glue along the vein of the eyelash
and wait for it to go tacky (about 10
seconds). Then, using tweezers or
your fingers, attach the lashes to your
natural lash line and hold in place for
a couple of seconds – this is the time
to make any adjustments.

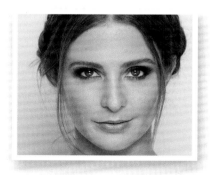

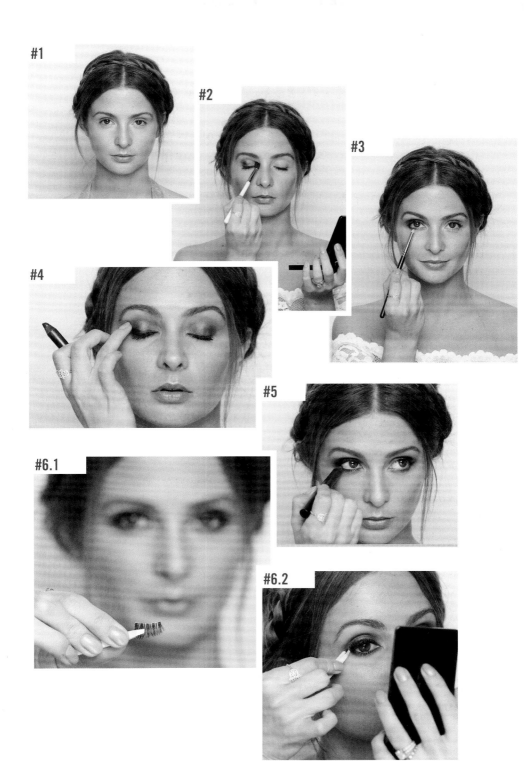

ADDING HIGHLIGHTS

This isn't something that I would do every day, but for a special occasion I will add highlights to ensure my eyes and lips look larger and my entire face is given definition. I use a light illuminating or sculpting powder for this. Dust very lightly; using your finger can be easier if you are trying this for the first time.

#1
Apply the Everyday Face (see pages 132–135).

#2
Lightly dot over your brow bone and the inner corner of your eyes.

#3
Lightly dust the very tops of your cheekbones, just under the outer corners of your eyes.

#4
Very lightly dot down the entire centre of your nose.

#5
Dust a small amount in the centre of your Cupid's bow.

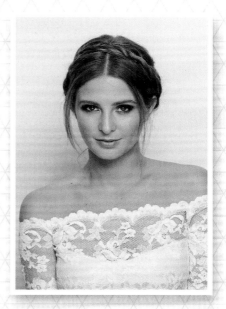

#1

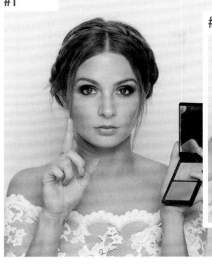

#2

#3

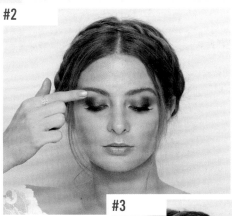

#4

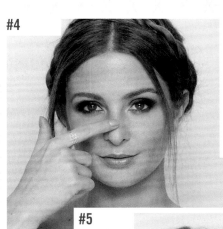

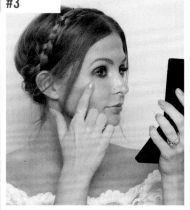

#5

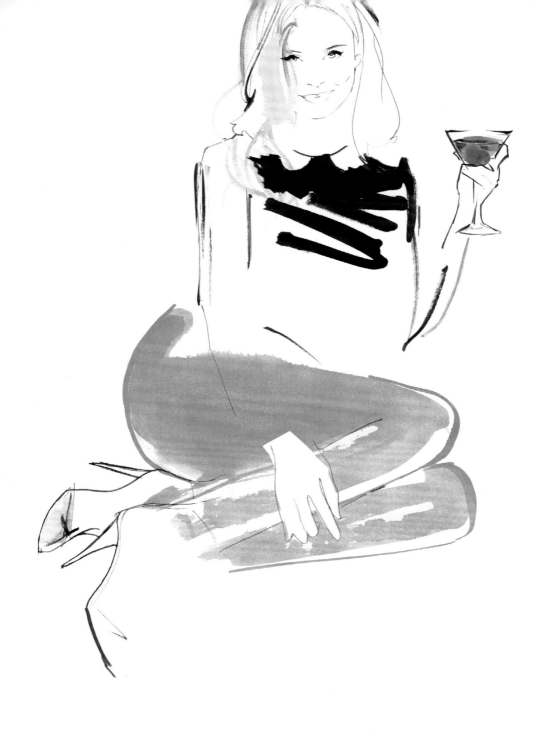

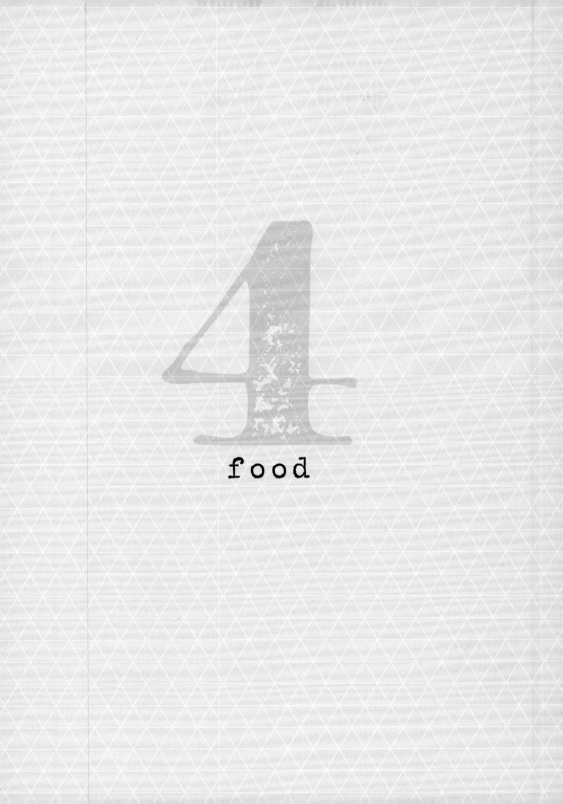

4
food

I love food. In fact, I think eating is my greatest pleasure in life. I grew up in a house that was always full of delicious, home-cooked dishes and being around my parents' delicatessen meant that I got used to strong flavours at an early age; I remember how toast smothered in Gentleman's Relish, made from anchovy paste, was one of my favourite things for breakfast. My sister and I used to help out in the shop kitchen too, and I was always nicking blocks of cheese when my dad wasn't looking. I still adore really smelly cheese.

These days I'm into fitness and I train hard, but I still love to cook tasty, filling meals. I'm a big fan of Italian cooking and one of my favourite dishes is *spaghetti alle vongole*, or spaghetti with clams. It's so simple and delicious and would probably be what I'd choose for my last meal on earth. Stephen and I picked the Almalfi Coast for our honeymoon largely because of the food – we had the most incredible Italian feast in this restaurant that you could only get to by boat. There wasn't a menu; you just ordered the catch of the day and they served it with some pasta. It was amazingly fresh.

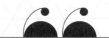

I think that eating is one of my greatest pleasures in life

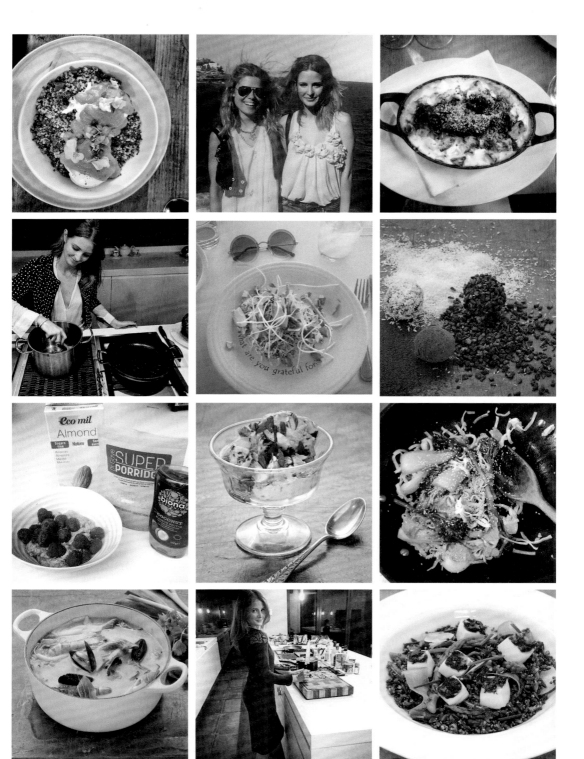

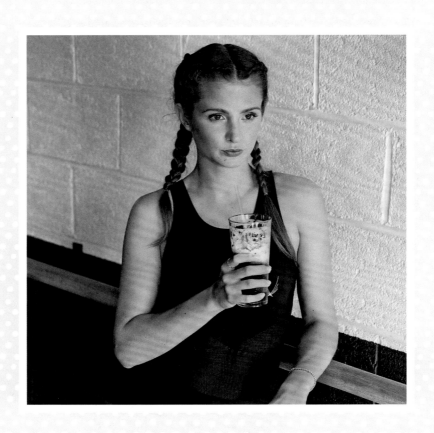

I got into exercise because I'd become 'skinny fat' (see page 20) – in other words, I had too little muscle and too much fat, all of which was stored on the inside, meaning that I was at greater risk of developing high blood pressure, high cholesterol and diabetes. Then, once I started working out, I realised that I wouldn't get maximum benefit from all the effort I was putting in at the gym unless I rethought my diet too. It wasn't that I lived entirely on takeaways and junk food, but I did eat whatever I fancied and that meant too much stodge, fat and sugar and too little veg. I needed guidance and so turned to the wonderful nutritional health coach Madeleine Shaw, who's also one of my best friends, and she helped me adopt a whole new way of eating. It's not a diet and it doesn't mean denying myself so that food loses all its pleasure (what kind of a life would that be?); no, the aim is to fuel my body with the right foods to keep me in optimum health and give me enough energy to exercise. What that means is avoiding processed food, refined sugar and certain carbohydrates, watching my intake of saturated fat and making gorgeous dishes that help keep me fit. It's an approach known as 'clean eating'. If it sounds a bit clinical, just think of it the other way round: do you want to eat 'dirty' food that is just junk or highly-processed foods? And, as you'll see from the recipes in this section, it's all about great-tasting, nutritious food that helps you look and feel energised and fantastic.

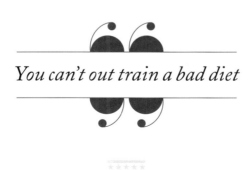

You can't out train a bad diet

CLEAN EATING
FOR EVERY DAY

I aim for an 70/30 clean diet because that's the balance of healthy to unhealthy food I need to maintain in order to achieve my personal goal – which is to be fit, not thin. The balance you choose for yourself may be different, depending on what your own aims are, but it goes without saying that the amount of good food you consume should outweigh the bad.

Basically, my clean way of eating is high in protein and vegetables and low in simple carbs. The protein helps to replenish lost energy reserves and restore muscle tissue, enabling me to recover and continue to train on a regular basis. Simple carbohydrates, found in table sugar, fruit juice and processed wheat products, are the sugars that raise your blood pressure quickly but have little nutritional value, so replacing them with complex carbs that take longer for the body

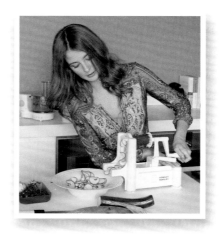

to digest means that you stay feeling full for longer and avoid the sugar rushes that tip the body out of balance and bring on horrible cravings.

Switching to this way of eating wasn't easy. Fibre-rich, complex carbohydrates like pulses, whole grains and vegetables are delicious, but at first I really missed processed wheat products like white pasta and I was longing for a sweet treat. (I used to have three teaspoons of sugar in my tea.) Allowing myself to have a full English breakfast, a bowl of pasta and a dessert at the weekend certainly helped, but I also found alternative ways to satisfy my weekday cravings and I trained myself off junk food by looking at the grease and the fat and the lurid colour of the ingredients and imagining the kitchen where it was made and then thinking, 'I'm putting that into my body.' It was a real turn-off.

Working with trainers helped me to keep going, but it was seeing and feeling the changes in my body that really spurred me on. Within weeks, I noticed that not only was I looking leaner, but I felt better too. My concentration levels improved, I was more alert and I had more energy. And the cravings stopped. A few weeks into this new eating lifestyle, I can honestly say that it felt completely normal to reach for a chai-seed pot rather than a piece of cake when my energy levels dipped and I became much more aware of planning my day to make sure that I was getting the right food and at the right time so my hunger levels didn't get too high. It's hard to make a sensible eating decision when you're hungry.

My working week isn't nine to five, Monday to Friday, but I try to eat clean on those days because, although it does mean thinking ahead and preparing meals in advance, there are fewer temptations during the week and keeping busy is a great distraction. It also allows me to eat whatever I fancy at the weekend – which is normally cheese and seafood spaghetti!

INGREDIENTS

I like to shop locally and always buy my meat, shellfish and fish from a sustainable source. I go to a butcher at the nearby farmers' market because I like to buy grass-fed, British red meat that hasn't travelled too far. It is more expensive than buying meat from the supermarket, but I'd always choose quality over quantity; no one needs to eat meat every day. I do a lot of slow roasts and casseroles, too, which are perfect for the cheaper cuts of meat such as shoulders of lamb or stewing steak.

I buy my veg from the farmers' market too – I grew up in the countryside and I remember pulling carrots and potatoes out of the ground. They looked weird with all the knobbly bits on them, but they tasted amazing. We're used to seeing perfect-looking vegetables, but I think you get a better taste from locally produced, seasonally grown food.

I'm lucky that we have a farmers' market and a branch of Whole Foods nearby, but I go to the supermarket too, of course. I don't shop online very much because I prefer to choose the food I'll be eating – that way I can buy what looks fresh rather than having to decide beforehand. If your local supermarket doesn't sell the kind of vegetables or healthy snacks that you're looking for, then you can have a box delivered. Abel & Cole, Riverford, Graze, Gousto, Hello Fresh or a local farm shop are all great options. And they even deliver recipe cards along with the ingredients.

THE CLEAN FRIDGE AND FREEZER

The 'clean' contents of my fridge and freezer varies with the seasons, of course, but all of the following will be there at some point in the year. Items with asterisks by them (and in the store cupboard list that follows) are foods that I use only sparingly during the week.

★ Almond milk
★ Apples
★ Asparagus
★ Aubergines
★ Avocados
★ Beef – fillet steak, mince, shin
★ Blueberries
★ Bok choy
★ Broccoli
★ Butter*
★ Carrots
★ Cauliflower
★ Cheese* – cottage, feta, halloumi
★ Chicken (free-range) – whole chicken, skinless and boneless breasts and thighs
★ Chilli peppers
★ China Rose radish sprouts
★ Clams
★ Courgettes
★ Damsons
★ Eggs (free-range)

★ Fish – salmon (fresh and smoked), white fillets such as cod, haddock, seabass or monkfish
★ Goose or duck fat*
★ Green beans
★ Herbs (fresh) – chives, coriander, lemon grass oregano, parsley, thyme, Vietnamese mint
★ Kale
★ King prawns
★ Lettuce – iceberg, Little Gem, romaine, round
★ Mangoes
★ Mascarpone
★ Mussels
★ Parsnips
★ Passion fruit
★ Pork and turkey mince
★ Portobello mushrooms, and other varieties of mushrooms
★ Radishes

- ★ Raspberries
- ★ Red cabbage
- ★ Rhubarb
- ★ Spring onions
- ★ Sugar snap peas
- ★ Swedes
- ★ Tofu
- ★ Tomatoes – beef, cherry
- ★ Watercress
- ★ Watermelon
- ★ Yoghurt (natural) – coconut (such as Co Yo), Greek*

I also have some packets of ready-marinated chicken or fish in there that I can pop straight in the oven when I'm busy. In the freezer I keep homemade stock and pots of chilli and meatballs in tomato sauce, along with dairy- and sugar-free ice cream (Booja Booja is delicious) and basics like frozen peas, spinach and berries.

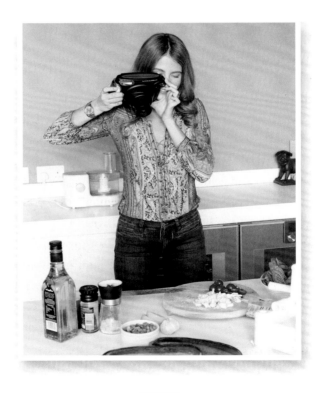

THE CLEAN STORE CUPBOARD

A store cupboard stocked with healthy basics means that a clean meal is possible even if the fridge is a little bare.

★ Agave syrup
★ Almond butter (unsweetened)
★ Almonds – flaked, ground
★ Anchovies (tinned)
★ Bananas
★ Bouillon stock powder – chicken, fish
★ Bulgur wheat*
★ Cacao powder (raw)
★ Capers
★ Chickpeas (tinned)
★ Chilli sauce
★ Chipotle chillies (dried)
★ Chocolate – dark (80% cocoa solids)*
★ Coconut chips
★ Coconut cream and milk
★ Coconut oil
★ Desiccated coconut
★ Désirée potatoes
★ Dried fruits – cranberries, dates, goji berries, prunes
★ Herbs (dried) – lime leaves, thyme
★ Fish sauce (nam pla)

★ Flour – buckwheat, rice
★ Garlic
★ Ginger root
★ Herbal teas
★ Honey or agave
★ Lemons – fresh (unwaxed), preserved
★ Limes
★ Kidney beans (tinned – sugar- and salt-free)
★ Maple syrup
★ Miso paste
★ Mung beans
★ Mushrooms (dried)
★ Mustard – Dijon, English
★ Noodles – buckwheat, rice
★ Nuts – cashews, hazelnuts, peanuts, pistachios, almonds
★ Olives
★ Oils – groundnut, olive (including extra-virgin), rapeseed, sesame seed
★ Onions – red, white, shallots
★ Pasta* – wholewheat, spelt
★ Polenta

- ★ Porridge oats (gluten-free)
- ★ Puy lentils
- ★ Quinoa – red, white
- ★ Quinoa flakes
- ★ Raspberry powder (freeze-dried)
- ★ Red rice
- ★ Rye bread
- ★ Sea salt
- ★ Seeds – chia, ground flaxseed, hemp, poppy, pumpkin, sesame
- ★ Soy sauce
- ★ Spelt
- ★ Spices – allspice, black and white pepper, cayenne pepper, chilli powder, cinnamon (both ground and sticks), coriander seeds, cumin seeds, dried chilli flakes, ground cardamom, star anise, sweet smoked paprika, turmeric
- ★ Stevia
- ★ Sugar – coconut, palm*
- ★ Sweetcorn (tinned)
- ★ Sweet potatoes
- ★ Tabasco sauce
- ★ Tahini
- ★ Tamari
- ★ Tomato purée
- ★ Tomatoes (tinned)
- ★ Vanilla extract
- ★ Tuna (tinned)
- ★ Vinegar – apple cider, red wine, rice
- ★ Wheat bran (organic)*
- ★ Wine (for cooking)* – red, white
- ★ Yeast flakes (deactivated)

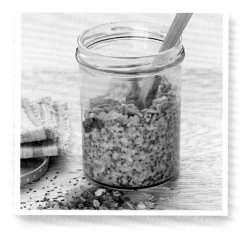

CLEAN BASICS

As you will see from all the recipes in this chapter, my clean eating regime is about cutting down on wheat, dairy products and sugar, rather than total abstinence. And reducing the number of simple carbs and processed wheat and dairy products you consume is actually quite easy. Here are a few of my favourite clean alternatives for some of the basic foods.

BREAD

Wheat-free breads offer a delicious, high-fibre alternative to your standard loaf. I love ones made from 100 per cent rye, but lots of different varieties are available, so just experiment until you find one you like. The 'free from' shelves of health-food shops and supermarkets are good places to find them, along with wheat-free flours for making your own bread. Do make sure that you check the ingredients, however – being wheat-free doesn't automatically mean they don't contain sugar or salt, for example.

If you make your own bread, try adding a few tablespoons of chia seeds to your standard recipe. (Just always remember to soak them overnight in water first.) The seeds will give your loaf extra protein and fibre. And if you want to avoid bread altogether, try lettuce leaves as a wrapping for a burger or falafel; they make a lovely low-carb alternative to rolls and tortillas.

BUTTER

I prefer to use a small amount of grass-fed butter rather than a low-fat spread on bread and vegetables, not only because it tastes better but because it contains lots of fat-soluble vitamins, including A, E and K_2. I'm not going to make a big deal out of A and E, because if you're eating a healthy diet that includes meat, fruit and vegetables, then you are probably getting enough of those already. However, vitamin K$_2$ is fairly rare in the modern diet and many people don't know about its powerful effects on health. It is intimately involved in calcium metabolism and a low intake has been associated with a number of serious conditions, including cardiovascular disease, cancer and osteoporosis.

I like to cook with coconut oil, which contains medium chain triglycerides, fatty acids that convert easily into energy rather than being stored as fat. (It also doubles as a great moisturiser!) However, this oil is not right for every recipe because it does leave a slight coconut flavour, so I like to ring the changes with rapeseed, olive or groundnut oil.

CHEESE

I love cheese but I do try to limit my dairy intake. This is partly because I cut out dairy completely for a while when I came back from my gap year – I was suffering from fatigue and omitting dairy products made me feel better – and partly because many products are highly processed. And they are high in fat too. Here are a few low-calorie or dairy-free alternatives:

★ Opt for cheese made with sheep or goat's milk such as feta and halloumi, which are lower in fat and more easily digested if you have an intolerance to cow's milk.
★ Try cottage cheese, made from pasteurised skimmed milk.
★ Make some cashew cheese. Simply soak 135g of cashews in water for 4 hours, then blend until smooth with the juice of half a lemon, 4 tablespoons of water, 2 cloves of garlic, 1 tablespoon of Dijon mustard, a pinch of salt and 1 tablespoon of apple cider vinegar. Yummy and, because cashew nuts are a great source of both

magnesium, which helps relax muscles, and vitamin K, which
is brilliant for getting rid of bags under your eyes, it's super
good for you too. I like it on its own or spooned over some
roasted vegetables, and you can use it to make cheese sauce too.

★ Deactivated yeast flakes – these taste and smell really cheesy
and can just be sprinkled over dishes, as you would Parmesan.

MILK

I use almond milk not only because it's dairy free but because it
has fewer calories than cow's milk and is loaded with skin-boosting
vitamin E. Also, unlike some dairy-free milks, it doesn't separate
in tea and can be used for every smoothie recipe you can think of.
Hemp and oat milk are readily available dairy substitutes too. Check
the ingredients list before you buy, however, as some dairy-free milk
contain added sugar. For pouring over a bowl of muesli I like to use
Co Yo coconut yoghurt instead of milk. I also have coconut yoghurt
with some fresh fruit as a snack.

PASTA

To avoid standard white pasta, a processed wheat product that is full
of simple carbs (see page 152), I substitute with spelt or wholewheat
pasta, which is higher in fibre, or with buckwheat noodles, which
contain fewer calories.

In addition, I love 'courgetti' noodles (see page 199 and 197), which
I make with my spiraliser. You just feed in a courgette and out come
long strips of courgetti. It doesn't taste like pasta, of course, but it
contains around a tenth of the calories and ups your veggie intake for
the day. The noodles also take on the flavour of sauces really well and
you can twist it round your fork it the same, comforting way.

POTATOES

As a low-calorie substitute for mashed potatoes, why not try cauliflower mash? Cauliflower is a real superfood: rich in antioxidants and other anti-inflammatory nutrients, it also contains a sulphur compound that has been linked to killing cancerous stem cells. Simply steam one chopped up head of cauliflower and purée with salt, a teaspoon of smoked paprika and a teaspoon of coconut oil. Sweet potatoes contain a bit more fibre and slightly fewer calories than standard spuds, as well as being higher in vitamins A and C. Cut into wedges and roasted with a little olive oil, they make delicious chips to accompany a steak or that mushroom bun burger (see page 205). Other root vegetables, such as carrots, parsnips and even swedes, are also brilliant roasted.

RICE

Nutritious, high-fibre grains like quinoa, bulgur wheat and spelt all make brilliant substitutes for white rice, which is more highly processed and therefore stripped of fibre and many nutrients. Spelt risotto is a real treat, for instance. Pulses such as lentils, kidney beans and chickpeas are comforting, filling and high in protein too. A vegetarian staple, pulses can also be used to add texture and flavour to meat dishes like stews and casseroles.

SUGAR

This is what Madeleine Shaw, my nutritional health coach, author of *Get the Glow* and one of my best friends, has to say about sugar.

Sugar is bad news. It's a simple carbohydrate with lots of calories but few nutrients. When we eat sugar, our energy levels rise almost instantly, but the spike is short-lived and before long we're back where we started. Too many sugar-fuelled energy rushes upset our natural blood-sugar levels and send our bodies off kilter, leaving us exhausted and craving another instant hit.

Unfortunately, sugar is abundant in so much processed food, not just in the obvious sweet treats. It's hidden in everything from breads and yoghurts to condiments – and even in supposedly healthy low-fat foods, compensating for the lack of flavour-giving fat. But with a bit of effort it's simple to avoid sugar. Start by checking the list of ingredients on the food you buy. The nearer to the top of the list an ingredient is, the more of it there is in that particular item.

Most soft drinks are loaded with sugar. Fizzy drinks are some of the worst offenders: in 2014, Action on Sugar found that 79 per cent of the sugary drinks included in its survey of 232 sugar-sweetened drinks from leading supermarkets contained at least 6 tablespoons of sugar per 330ml can. Don't be seduced by the sugar-free alternatives, either; they contain fake-sugar substitutes, which upset your metabolism because, by ingesting this sweet calorie-free liquid, you're telling your body to expect a hit of sugar but no energy actually arrives, so the craving remains unsatisfied.

Fruit juice is high in sugar too. We're all brought up to think that it's good for you, but in fact a glass of orange juice probably has five oranges in it – which equates to the most ridiculous amount of sugar. You're much better off eating whole fruit (go for two portions a day of low-sugar varieties such as raspberries, strawberries or watermelon) or drinking a fresh 'green' juice made with two part vegetables to one part fruit. One a day is sufficient.

If you find drinking water boring, add a bit of cucumber to it, or a sprig of mint. I love to drink it hot, spiced up with some fresh lemon juice (see page 165) or a few mint leaves. Coconut water is another option; it's a bit of an acquired taste, but it's good for the digestion and people say that it lowers blood pressure and cures hangovers too!

TIPS TO QUIT SUGAR

I know that sugar tastes good and that most of us have an emotional relationship with it, but I have devised 6 tips to help you break the habit:

#1 EAT BREAKFAST

Missing meals leads to a dip in blood-sugar levels, causing cravings. Start the day with a nice healthy breakfast like poached eggs with avocado and salmon.

#2 UP YOUR PROTEIN INTAKE

Eating protein-rich foods such as fish, chicken, quinoa or eggs will keep you feeling full and help reduce your desire for sugar.

#3 ADD FLAVOUR

Sweeten your coffee with a pinch of cinnamon and a drop of vanilla extract.

#4 REDUCE STRESS

Reduce stress – sugar cravings are linked to your stress levels, so run a bath, take a yoga class (see page 274) or do some belly breathing. (For more on stress relief, see pages 277–281.)

#5 SWITCH TO A NATURAL SUGAR ALTERNATIVE

With a low GI and high mineral and vitamin content, coconut sugar makes a healthier alternative to standard cane sugar. It has a gorgeous caramel taste too – you could swap it for the same quantity of sugar in your favourite cake recipe. Stevia, a carb-free natural sweetener, is another great sugar substitute. Use it in powdered form, as you would cane sugar, but be aware that stevia is about four times as sweet as cane sugar, so you need to adjust the quantities accordingly. Dishes such as porridge and yoghurt can be sweetened with a few chopped or puréed dates.

#6 ADJUST YOUR SUPPLEMENTS

Take chromium, which helps regulate blood-sugar levels and prevents the dips you get from eating sugary food.

MILLIE'S CLEAN MEALS

BREAKFAST

Every day begins with a mug of hot water mixed with the juice of half a lemon. The surprising thing about lemons is that although they taste acidic, they actually have an alkalising effect on your digestive system. Foods like red meat and tomatoes cause acidity when you eat them, so a drink of lemon water will restore the natural balance, help to cleanse the body and fire up your digestive system ready for breakfast. (Just remember to add the lemon to lukewarm, rather than boiling, water, which will kill the enzymes.) I've recently started adding a tablespoon of apple cider vinegar to my lemon juice and water, too, because it's considered an alkaliser and is also meant to help burn fat. (There's a diet that involves drinking a tablespoon of apple cider vinegar half an hour before every meal. If you're not keen on the taste, just down it like a shot.) I don't like to eat the same thing every morning, so here are four of my favourite breakfasts.

★ *Instant oat, chia & sunflower seed porridge (see page 186)*
★ *Smashed avocado & dukkah-rolled eggs on rye toast (see page 188)*
★ *Egg-white & spinach omelette with smoked salmon (see page 187)*
★ *Cauliflower & corn fritters (see page 190)*

LUNCH

I try to eat my complex carbs at lunch, rather than in the evening, so I can burn off the energy during the afternoon. These are some of the dishes I like to make when I'm at home.

★ *Miso-glazed tofu quinoa & red rice lunch bowl (see page 192)*
★ *Green gazpacho with toasted tamari pumpkin seeds & feta*
  (see page 194)
★ *Cheat's pho (see page 191)*
★ *Spice-crusted chicken with sweet potato & tomato salad (see page 196)*
★ *Cold buckwheat noodles with crispy ginger & chilli pork (see page 198)*
★ *Wild garlic pesto with raw courgetti (see page 197)*

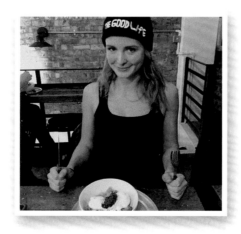

LUNCH ON THE GO

Of course, most people are out at work at lunchtime. I worked in an office when I was interning at Glamour and Grazia magazines, and every day I'd go to Starbucks and buy a ham and cheese croissant for breakfast with a chai tea latte and a bit of sugar. By mid-morning, I'd have a headache and be starving, so I'd go to Itsu and buy enough for three lunches – noodle soup, a large packet of sushi rolls, a load of snacks and a sugary drink. Terrible! Yet it's not impossible to eat clean when your work is office-based or you are travelling a lot. Here are some ideas:

 # FILL UP WITH PROTEIN RATHER THAN CARBOHYDRATES. Lots of places are now doing healthier options and the chains on the high street are improving, so you are no longer restricted to just sandwiches and crisps. Salads and protein bars fill you up as well as being full of flavour and if you need a quick snack, try a protein pot, such as boiled eggs and tuna. (Pret A Manger do some good ones now.)

 # GO JAPANESE. Japanese food is very clean and readily available now. (Just watch out for sushi rice because it's made with lots of sugar and salt; brown rice sushi is better for you.) My favourites are seaweed salad, broths made with rice noodles, and plain edamame beans.

 # MAKE YOUR OWN. Tupperware may not seem very cool at first, but homemade lunches are tastier, healthier and cheaper than bought alternatives. You can buy some great, sturdy containers nowadays. These are all easy to fill with meat, veg or grains from the previous evening's meal – just remember to make extra, with lunch in mind. They travel well too.

SUPPER

My mum once told me that you should always see more than one colour on your plate. It's good advice if you're aiming for a well-balanced diet and following it doesn't mean that you have to make a complicated meal every night. You can knock up a delicious, healthy dish with plenty of veg and protein in only half an hour. (I try to keep weekday suppers pretty much carb-free because carbohydrates just sit in your stomach overnight.) I also like to make something more time-consuming such as meatballs in a tomato sauce or chilli at the weekend and freeze it in single portions. Then all I have to do on a weeknight is stick it the microwave. The following are all regulars in my house.

★ *Coconut & quinoa seafood soup (see page 200)*
★ *Courgetti with clams, cherry tomatoes & chilli (see page 199)*
★ *Pan-roasted salmon, shaved broccoli & green beans with tahini-poppy seed dressing (see page 202)*
★ *Baked aubergines with tomatoes, feta & thyme (see page 204)*
★ *Vietnamese chicken meatballs with mango, chilli & spring onion salsa (see page 206)*
★ *Mushroom bun burgers with halloumi (see page 205)*
★ *Melting beef with cauliflower rice (see page 209)*
★ *Seared beef with chimichurri & sweet potato chips (see page 211)*

CLEAN PUDDINGS

Eating clean doesn't mean missing out on puddings. The following are both healthy, easy to throw together and completely delicious.

★ *Overnight chia & almond milk pudding (see page 212)*
★ *Homemade pink fro-yo (see page 213)*

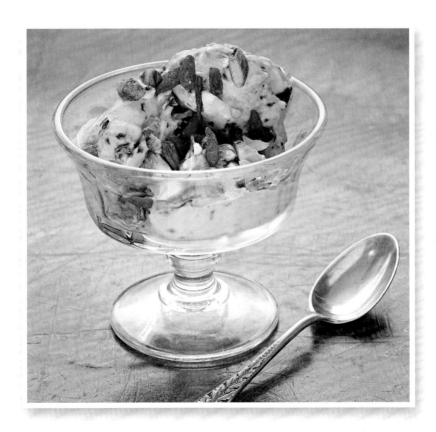

EATING CLEAN & ENTERTAINING

Eating clean doesn't have to mean avoiding supper parties. I love having friends over for meals. Presentation makes all the difference and I learned some great tricks when I appeared on *MasterChef*. These are my top tips:

Always use odd numbers for a garnish, e.g. one or three raspberries.

Garnishes look much better when they shine, so rub those micro herbs in a bit of olive oil.

A dusting of icing sugar turns plain fruit into a posh dessert.

Artistic smears across the plate look cheffy and are easy to do; just use a spatula, squeezy bottle or a piping bag with a small nozzle.

Use big plates – the rim of the plate should always stay clean.

Always serve pasta in a bowl.

Try and make a tower with your food. On *MasterChef*, I cut the calves' livers in half to add height.

I like to plan the lighting, music and colour theme too. Create an ambiance with scented candles and keep the dimmers turned low. The colour scheme in my house is mostly black, white and shades of grey, so I wouldn't choose a heavy headache of colours for the table. I like to keep it simple with lots of fresh flowers – I have low vases of roses on the table that look lovely but don't block people's view.

I think about the seating plan as well. It's nice to put guests together who haven't met before, but be considerate – don't sit someone who's teetotal next to a heavy drinker, for example. And get everyone to move around in between courses.

MIDWEEK SUPPER
WITH THE GIRLS

These days, my girlfriends and I are so busy trying to carve out
careers that we don't have time to see each other as much as we'd
like, so it's super-important that we get together and have a good
girly gossip every month. And there's no better way to do that than
round the kitchen table. We take turns to host and sometimes
everyone brings a dish along so it's more like a supper club. We
do try to eat clean at these evenings – we all want to look good,
after all, so why not make a delicious meal that's also guilt free?

My go-to dish for supper with my girlfriends would be
homemade flaxseed crackers and tapenade for a starter, roast
chicken for the main, followed by a bought-in dessert like ice
cream (preferably sugar and dairy free).

★ *Superseed crackers with black olive tapenade*
  (see page 214)
★ *Lemony roast chicken (see page 216)*
★ *Stephen's roast potatoes (see page 217)*

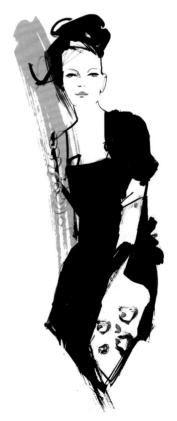

FULL-BLOWN SUNDAY LUNCH WITH FRIENDS

I don't usually do formal dinner parties but Sunday lunch has become a bit of an institution at our house. And full blown it certainly is: these meals are a celebration of the fact that we're getting a group of people together around a table – and enjoy it we do. Calories do not matter and I can eat what I fancy as it's the weekend! The following combination of dishes would be my top favourite. It includes my fail-safe dessert, Damson Ripple Roulade, which I did on MasterChef and which I make with my mum's delicious homemade damson purée.

★ *Slow-roast pork belly with red cabbage & cranberries (see page 218)*
★ *Damson ripple roulade (see page 220)*

Mum's gravy

When roasting a joint of meat, always cook on top of onions, celery or carrots, to add flavour. Once cooked, remove the meat from the pan, cover with foil and set aside to rest for 20 minutes. Meanwhile:

★ Skim off any excess fat from the pan, leaving the juices. Place the pan on top of the hob over a moderate heat and add one dessertspoon of plain flour. Scrape the bottom of the pan with a wooden spoon, releasing all the burnt gooey bits (this is where the flavour is) and mix the flour and the meat juices together. The mixture will look lumpy at this stage, but don't worry – it'll come together.

★ Take the pan off the heat and add half a glass of red or white wine, stirring all the time, then pour in 300ml of homemade or vegetable stock. Place back on the heat and slowly bring to the boil, stirring all the while. Season with salt and pepper and let the gravy boil for a few minutes to reduce a little. Taste, adding a little Marmite or Bovril for colour and saltiness, then strain the gravy into a serving jug.

STRESS-FREE ENTERTAINING

Cooking for other people can be stressful, though it shouldn't be. These are your friends, after all! These are my top tips for relaxed entertaining:

#1

Cook something you have made before and pretty much cooks itself – I love slow roasts you can just stick in the oven (see the recipe on pages 218–219 and some tips on making gravy opposite). I have had a couple of disasters cooking joints of meat I haven't done before. One was a massive piece of beef that just wouldn't cook. We ended up cutting it up and flash-frying it …

#2

Go for a cold pudding, one that can be made in advance, like my Damson Ripple Roulade (see page 220), and keep it in the fridge/freezer until you're ready to serve.

#3

Put some music on, open some booze. Sunday roasts at our place always start with a glass of champagne or prosecco.

#4

Have a rough plan of when you want food to be ready.

#5

If you are cooking with your partner or a friend, decide in advance what your jobs will be and stick to them.

#6

Get the guests to help with peeling the veg and laying the table.

#7

Don't feel the pressure to make everything yourself – I've served fruit and shop-bought ice cream for pudding on many an occasion and had no complaints.

#8

Remember, if it all goes wrong you can always order a takeaway – this is the weekend, after all.

BAKING

Baking is something that brings back childhood memories of cooking with my mum (she would send me to primary school every Monday with brownies for the teachers) and it still fills me with joy. There's nothing better than chatting with a friend over a slice of cake. In recent years I have adapted my diet so that I eat less sugar, but I do still eat full-fat, sugary cake as a treat at the weekend. And if I'm having people to stay, I always make sure there's homemade cake in the house just in case they come down for a midnight snack. My guests never go hungry. Here are three brilliant bakes that won't spend a lifetime on your hips:

★ *Lemon polenta & almond cake (see page 225)*
★ *Banana & bran muffins with roasted rhubarb jam (see page 221)*
★ *Nutty butter & seed cookies (see page 224)*

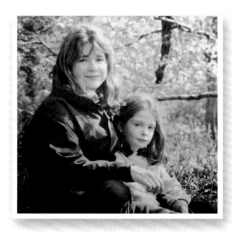

ALCOHOL

I read somewhere that one margarita has the same amount of calories as a cheeseburger! Margaritas are my favourite cocktails, so that certainly came as a shock. Up until then, I'd never really thought about how many calories there were in alcoholic drinks, but now I know, I limit my drinking to two nights a week, ideally at the weekend. I'm too much of a foodie to waste loads of calories on drink. Plus I think it's a good idea to give your liver a chance to recover before drinking again.

When I do drink, I like tequila with soda water or gin and slimline tonic, both with lots of ice and lime, or classic champagne cocktails with brandy-soaked sugar cubes, like my grandfather used to make. (One is enough; any more and chaos will ensue!) I grew up with parents who had a shop specialising in wonderful food and drink so I will happily share a bottle of full-bodied red wine over a meal and, in my opinion, nothing beats a pale rosé on a warm sunny evening.

*I'm far too much of
a foodie to waste my calories
on an alcoholic drink!*

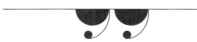

PARTIES

Parties are tricky if you're trying to eat clean. You may decide to have a night off (and I quite often do), but if you want to stick to the plan, here are my top three survival tips:

#1

Don't arrive hungry. A friend once told me that a good way to look at hunger is in levels from one to ten, ten being ravenous. If you arrive at a party at level ten, then you'll just dive straight into the canapés, so eat something beforehand to take you down to around level five.

#2

Be selective with the canapés. I either avoid bread-based nibbles like sandwiches and mini burgers or, if I'm lucky enough to have been given a plate, I take the meat out of the bun.

#3

Choose your drink wisely. Prosecco has fewer calories that champagne, red wine less than white. Sugary mixers can be swapped for soda or slimline tonic, or left out completely.

hangovers

There are two ways to treat a hangover: indulge or cure. The first – indulging your hangover by spending the day on the sofa and feeding it with all the nasty things it's craving – is fine, and I must admit to spending quite a lot of Sundays doing just that, but sometimes we have to function the morning after the night before. These are some good cures:

★ Tomatoes – either as juice (no vodka!) or as a meal. Baked eggs in tomato sauce make a great morning-after breakfast
★ Coconut water
★ Watermelon
★ Rehydration sachet

EATING CLEAN
FOR FITNESS

Someone once told me that 'abs are made in the kitchen'. And it's true: in order to fine-tune your body, you can't just go to the gym: you have to look at what you're eating too. That's where most of the change is going to come from.

Eating clean for fitness is all about putting the right fuel in your body. I soon realised that there's no point in putting lots of effort in at the gym if you go and get a MacDonald's straight after training. It's tempting to think, 'Oh, I've just exercised so I can get away with eating whatever I want.' But while maybe you can, calorie-wise, I've learned that you will only see results if you're also fuelling your body with the right things. If you're training hard, then you need food with lots of nutrients and enough protein to allow your muscles to repair properly between sessions. I've picked up masses of tips from fitness trainers, many of whom are trained in nutrition, and this is what works for me.

PRE-WORKOUT

What and when I eat on training days depends on when I'm working out. If I have a session first thing in the morning, then I won't eat anything beforehand – it's not good to train on a full stomach and training on empty is more effective because you start the day having burned a load of calories that you haven't actually eaten. So, if I'm training at 8 a.m., I'll wake up at 7.30 and have a black coffee (no sugar!), which usually kills any hunger pangs until afterwards. It's important to listen to your own body, though, and if you are just starting out on a training programme, it's probably a good idea to have something light and high in protein beforehand until you are used to it. A handful of nuts or a protein shake would be good. (Top tip: making a shake up the night before and leaving it in the fridge saves valuable time in bed.) It's important to avoid sugar because you want to burn fat in the gym not a load of sugar calories.

POST-WORKOUT

Before I got in to fitness, I thought protein shakes were for bodybuilders, but these days I often have one straight after a workout. The protein is absorbed really quickly so your body gets what it's craving straight away. My favourite is made with a rice-based protein powder – banana and vanilla – that I mix with coconut water to rehydrate me. Bananas are sugary and carby, both of which I need when I've sweated out lots of salt and sugar. This tastes just like a milk shake.

Protein shakes are NOT meal replacements (and you shouldn't have more than one per day), so it's important to eat a proper meal containing equal quantities of protein, carbohydrates and vegetables within an hour of a workout – especially if you didn't eat beforehand. I will often take a container filled with sweet potato, salmon and broccoli that I've made the night before to eat at the gym. The morning workout means that I can definitely afford some carbs.

SUPPER

I usually have chicken or salmon with a steamed veg salad for supper because I try to avoid white carbs in the evening. I'll add pulses or grains to make it more filling. I avoid creamy dressings but I love balsamic vinegar and citrus juice.

SNACKS

Working out makes you hungry. As I consume about 2,000 calories, or sometimes slightly less, on a training day (that happens to be the recommended daily allowance for women, but calorie intake depends on your size, age and level of physical activity, so what's right for you may be different), I need some snacks between my three main meals. I prefer savoury things, so kale or vegetable crisps and seaweed crisps from Itsu (and now available in Waitrose) are my favourites. If you have more of a sweet tooth, then try a chia seed pudding or Co Yo yoghurts, which are dairy and sugar free and contain a natural sweetener called xylitol that helps you fight that sweet craving. Add some berries, too, for extra goodness. Fruit is good, but you need to be aware that it contains a lot of sugar in the form of fructose. I try to stick to low-sugar fruits such as blueberries or raspberries.

Protein bites, protein balls and date balls are all good for energy. Dark chocolate is OK too. (If you're not keen on the bitter taste, then go for bars made with coconut milk – you can find them in health-food shops.) I love chocolate, especially if it has nuts or berries in it, but I find it hard to resist if I know it's in the house, so I buy those little Green & Black's bars. Every once in a while, however, I make some homemade truffles for an indulgent treat.

★ *Coconut, cardamom & bitter chocolate truffles (see page 226)*

DETOXING

Our bodies are designed to get rid of toxins naturally, so there is some debate about whether or not it's worth following a detox programme at all. I believe that there are times when my body needs a bit of extra help – I always need one after a boozy period like Christmas or a holiday in Ibiza, for example. The telltale signs are bloating, dull congested skin, weight gain and general tiredness.

What constitutes a detox varies hugely. For some, it's simply a day or two without coffee or alcohol, while for others it's a fortnight of juices. (If you are thinking about setting out on an intense detox, then it's important to seek medical advice first.) I like to use a detox to kick-start a healthier eating regime when things have slipped. When I'm detoxing, I drink aloe vera juice as it's really cleansing for the digestive system – I just add a few drops to my daily smoothie every day.

These are all things you might like to detox from:

★ Alcohol
★ Caffeine
★ Dairy products
★ Fatty foods
★ Gluten-containing products like wheat-based bread and pasta
★ Red meat
★ Refined sugar found in sweets, cakes and pastries
★ Salty, processed food

TIPS FOR DETOXING

#1

Doing a detox doesn't mean becoming a total hermit, but as it does involve a bit of self-control, it will be a lot easier if you choose a time when life is quiet. Also, you might well feel tired and emotional during the detox and skin breakouts are quite common (the results are worth it, honestly!), so this isn't a time to be partying.

#2

Clear all the food you're detoxing from out of the house – after all, why make it more difficult for yourself?

#3

Try to eat at home as much as possible. If you have to eat out, make sure you choose where you go, or head to a juice bar where you can have something without breaking your detox routine. The Good Life Eatery, with branches in Chelsea and Marylebone, is one of my favourites.

#4

Prepare your body by drinking more water, avoiding alcohol and sugar-rich foods and increasing your intake of the sorts of food you will be eating during the cleanse.

#5

Plan nice things to do during the detox, like a yoga class with a friend.

#6

Plan a treat for when you're done – pamper days are good. (You may think that you'll want a meal out, but be careful: your body will need to readjust to normal eating.)

DETOX ROUTINES

There are lots of different detox routines and you need to choose one that suits you and your lifestyle. Here are my top three, with web addresses for further details:

 # CHRIS JAMES MIND AND BODY CLEANSE – a 12-day detox in four phases, including three juice-only days. The pack includes a full detox kit and menu guide: www.chrisjamescleanse.com

 # HONESTLY HEALTHY CLEANSE – a book by Honestly Healthy's Natasha Corrett containing guides to four different cleanses, Feel Good, Slimdown, High Energy and Life Changing: www.honestlyhealthyfood.com

 # PURIFYNE CLEANSE – a juice-only cleanse available in packs lasting three, five, seven, nine or 14 days. The pack is more expensive than the one for the Chris James routine but contains everything you need: www.purifynecleanse.com

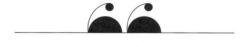

Detoxing does require some self-control, so it will be easier if you choose a time when life is quieter

PRE-HOLIDAY EATING PLAN

I want to look super-toned on holiday. Ideally, I would have been working out and following my clean-eating regime for weeks beforehand, but life isn't always like that and sometimes I need to get a bit strict with myself for a week in the run-up to going away. That means eating clean at the weekends too and reducing my carb intake a bit more than usual. I replace the carbs with protein so that I have enough energy to train hard, and really pile leafy greens onto my plate. You can never have enough broccoli, girls! This is my plan.

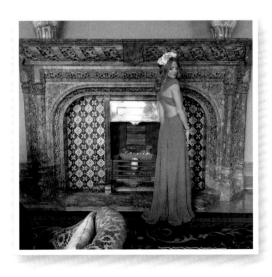

BASIC RULES

★ Eat little and often. This is the key to getting through the fortnight. You need at least six small meals a day and you shouldn't go too long without eating because you'll need energy in order to train!

★ Cut out all alcohol.

★ Cut out sugar.

★ Cut out all fried and processed foods.

★ Cut back on carbs. You don't have to stop eating carbohydrate completely but you do need to have the right ones at the right time – I only eat a small amount of carbs after exercising and eat healthy fats like avocado and nuts to keep my energy levels high.

★ Fill up with leafy greens.

★ Asparagus! Asparagus is a diuretic; it does make your pee smell funny, but it's brilliant at getting rid of bloating.

★ Aim for a lighter meal in the evening containing protein and vegetables or a salad.

FOODS TO EAT

These are all good, clean foods to eat during your pre-holiday plan:

★ Skinless chicken breast, turkey, lean fillet steak, fish of all kinds

★ Seasonings – I love chilli, ginger, garlic, lemon and soy sauce

★ Dark, leafy greens like kale, broccoli or spinach

★ Sweet potatoes (lunch only!)

★ Eggs – great for a quick breakfast and you can throw in some protein and vegetables to make a delicious omelette

★ Fruit-free green juice. I either have one for breakfast, a snack mid-morning, or at night just before I go to bed. The juice alkalises you (see page 165) and has a good effect on your body while you sleep. It also prevents hunger in the night.

CLEAN EATING FOR LIFE

I really hope that all the recipes, tips and suggestions in this chapter have shown that clean eating can be both healthy and delicious. There are some rules, but I find them helpful – I'm a glutton at heart and if I didn't have any rules in place, I would literally eat the earth – and I can honestly say that this way of eating has made look and feel better without taking all the pleasure out of food.

When I'm no longer modelling, I probably will be a bit more relaxed, but I really do see myself continuing to eat like this because I enjoy it. And if I fall off the wagon sometimes, which I do, I don't feel guilty (guilt is so destructive), because I know what to do to re-balance things. If I sound like a convert to the cause, it's because I am and I hope that the recipes here convince you too!

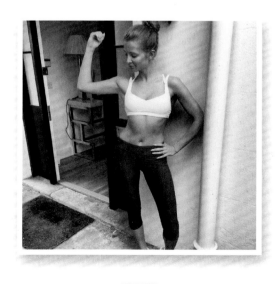

INSTANT OAT, CHIA & SUNFLOWER SEED PORRIDGE

This is your speedy midweek breakfast solution. Make a batch for the week ahead on Sunday (or at any time, for that matter), decant some into a mug, or transport in a jar, and all you need is some hot water from a kettle to have a healthy and sustaining breakfast on the go. Plus, it's porridge without the hassle of cleaning a pan.

PREP TIME: 2 MINUTES
MAKES: 5 SERVINGS (ENOUGH FOR 1 WORKING WEEK OF SPEEDY BREAKFASTS)

200g porridge oats
   (I use gluten-free ones)
60g chia seeds

Per mug/jar
1 tsp coconut oil
1 tsp sunflower seeds
1–2 tsp coconut or palm sugar
1 tbsp fresh berries, dried fruits or sliced banana (optional)

Pulse the oats lightly in a food processor (keep a chunky texture and be sure to not blend it to a powder as it will get gluey when you add water) and decant into an airtight plastic container or large jar to store for the week ahead. Measure the chia seeds into the container and shake them up to combine well.

On each weekday morning, add 50g of this mixture to your favourite mug (for eating in) or a clean, screw-top jam jar (for taking to go). Add the coconut oil, sunflower seeds and sugar to taste.

When you're ready to eat, pour boiling water from a kettle over the top (about 250ml – depending on how thick or thin you like your porridge), stir the mixture and leave it for 2 minutes to absorb and transform into your morning porridge. You can also add fresh berries, dried fruits, banana slices or whatever takes your fancy.

EGG-WHITE & SPINACH OMELETTE WITH SMOKED SALMON

Egg-white omelettes are airy and light, and definitely not just for the diet conscious. Not to be restricted to breakfast, these make a great speedy lunch or weekend brunch.

PREP TIME: 5 MINUTES
COOKING TIME: 5–10 MINUTES
MAKES: 2 OMELETTES

1 tbsp butter or rapeseed oil
8 egg whites
50g spinach
1 lemon
100g smoked salmon or
   smoked mackerel
sea salt

Heat the butter or oil in a small non-stick frying pan over a medium-low heat. While the pan is heating, whisk together four of the egg whites and a pinch of salt, incorporating a lot of air into the eggs as you whisk them to ensure the omelette is light and fluffy.

Pour the eggs into the hot frying pan and move the mixture from side to side to cover the base of the pan. Cook for 1–2 minutes or until the omelette has set, and then add half the spinach in a line down the middle. Use a spatula to flip over the sides of the omelette to cover the spinach, then slide the folded omelette onto a plate, seam side down. Repeat the same process to make the second omelette.

Cut the lemon in half and add one half to each plate. Lay the smoked salmon to the side of each omelette and serve.

SMASHED AVOCADO & DUKKAH-ROLLED EGGS ON RYE TOAST

This dukkah – a crunchy and fragrant spicy nut topping – is so versatile. It really peps up the eggs here, but goes with so many dishes otherwise: add it to salads, soups or dips. After storing, you can refresh the mix by dry-frying it again.

PREP TIME: 5 MINUTES
COOKING TIME: 5 MINUTES
MAKES: 2 SERVINGS

2 medium eggs
2 pieces of rye bread
1 avocado
1–2 tbsp fresh lemon juice
sea salt and black pepper

*For the hazelnut dukkah
(makes 100g)*
60g blanched hazelnuts
40g sesame seeds
2 tsp cumin seeds
2 tsp coriander seeds

To make the dukkah, place all the ingredients in a non-stick frying pan and toast over a medium-high heat for 2–3 minutes, shaking the pan frequently to prevent the nuts and seeds from burning. Allow to cool and then whizz in a food processor, or grind with a pestle and mortar. Season with salt and pepper to taste and store in an airtight plastic container or jar.

Place the eggs in a small saucepan and cover with cold water from the tap. Bring to the boil and cook for 3 minutes (for soft and oozy inside).

While the eggs are boiling, toast the rye bread and cut the avocado in half, removing the stone. Scoop the flesh out of each avocado half and smash in a bowl with a fork. Season with the lemon juice and salt and pepper to taste.

Remove the eggs from the heat and place in a bowl of cold water, then peel each egg and roll in the dukkah. Spread the avocado on each piece of toasted rye bread, place an egg on top and cut open to ooze onto the toast.

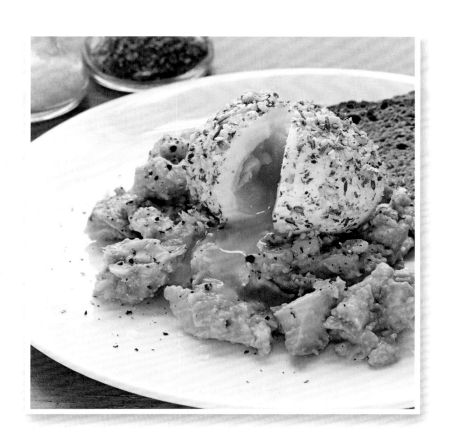

CAULIFLOWER & CORN FRITTERS

Gluten and dairy free, these super-speedy fritters have
a great little kick from the cayenne pepper.

PREP TIME: 10 MINUTES
COOKING TIME: 10 MINUTES
MAKES: 4 FRITTERS /
4 SERVINGS

100g cauliflower (about
 ¼ small head, stalk removed)
165g tinned sweetcorn
 (drained weight)
2 medium eggs
60g rice flour
20ml almond milk
½ tsp cayenne pepper
½ tsp sea salt
2 tbsp coconut oil
1 lime, quartered, to serve

Break the cauliflower florets into 1cm pieces and
place in a bowl with the drained sweetcorn. Break
the eggs into a separate bowl and add the rice
flour, almond milk, cayenne pepper and salt. Add
half of the cauliflower pieces and sweetcorn to
the wet ingredients and place in a food processor.
Blend until smooth and add to the remaining
sweetcorn and cauliflower in the bowl.

Melt half the coconut oil in a large non-stick
frying pan over a medium heat. Once the oil is
hot, add a large spoonful of fritter mixture and
then a second one, allowing plenty of space
between. (It's best to cook the fritters in two
batches to avoid crowding the pan.)

Cook the fritters for 2–3 minutes on one side,
then flip over and cook for a further 2–3 minutes
or until golden and not soft in the middle.
Remove from the pan and drain on kitchen paper.
Repeat the process to cook the remaining fritters.

Serve with a lime wedge on the side. These
fritters are delicious served with a poached egg
and a couple of slices of avocado, or with some
feta crumbled over.

CHEAT'S PHO

A traditional pho (Vietnamese noodle soup) is a labour of love.
My version is very much a quick alternative making use of the homemade stock I
keep in the freezer (though Bouillon stock powder is fine otherwise) and any
fresh veg I may have in the fridge. So feel free
to experiment and simply use this recipe as a guide.

PREP TIME: 5–10 MINUTES
COOKING TIME: 12 MINUTES
MAKES: 2 SERVINGS

750ml chicken or vegetable
stock
1 tsp coriander seeds
2 star anise
1 cinnamon stick
1 skinless and boneless chicken
breast (about 270g)
60g vermicelli or rice noodles
1 medium carrot, peeled and
cut into thin matchsticks
100g sugar snap peas, trimmed
juice of 1 lime
1 tsp sesame seed oil
1 tbsp tamari

To serve
China Rose radish sprouts
1 small (10g) bunch of
coriander or Vietnamese
mint

Pour the stock into a medium saucepan (with a
lid) set over a medium heat and add the coriander
seeds, star anise and cinnamon stick. Add the
chicken to the pan and press down to submerge
in the stock. Bring the stock to a simmer with
the lid on the pan and cook for 10 minutes.

After 10 minutes, add the vermicelli or rice
noodles, carrot matchsticks and sugar snap peas
and cook for 2 minutes or until the noodles are
soft. Remove the pan from the heat.

Take out the chicken and use two forks to shred it.
Return the shredded meat to the pan and add the
lime juice, sesame seed oil and tamari. Reheat the
soup if needed before dividing between two bowls
and garnishing with radish sprouts and the leaves
from the coriander or Vietnamese mint.

MISO-GLAZED TOFU QUINOA & RED RICE LUNCH BOWL

My lunch bowls are often a colourful medley of leftover vegetables and grains. One of my favourite grain combinations is a mix of red rice and quinoa, which I love for their texture and bite.

PREP TIME: 5–10 MINUTES
COOKING TIME: 35 MINUTES
MAKES: 4 SERVINGS

100g red rice
100g red quinoa
200g asparagus spears,
    cut into 5cm lengths
3 tbsp miso paste
1 tbsp rice vinegar
1 tbsp maple syrup
300g firm tofu
1 tbsp extra-virgin olive oil
1 tbsp fresh lemon juice
1 small (10g) bunch of chives,
    finely chopped, plus
    extra to garnish
4 medium carrots, peeled
4 radishes, thinly sliced
sea salt and black pepper

Bring a medium saucepan of salted water to the boil. Add the red rice, and simmer for 25 minutes, before adding the quinoa and cooking for a further 8–10 minutes. Drop the asparagus in for the last 2 minutes and drain everything in a sieve.

In the meantime, mix the miso paste in a small bowl with the rice vinegar and maple syrup.

While the rice and quinoa are cooking, preheat your grill to medium. Cut the tofu into 4cm x 4cm x 1cm pieces, place on a baking tray lined with foil and dollop or spread a teaspoon of miso paste on the top of each piece. Place under the grill to cook for 8–10 minutes or until lightly caramelised.

In a large bowl, toss the cooked rice, quinoa and asparagus with the olive oil, lemon juice and chives, seasoning with a pinch of salt and a few grinds of black pepper. Use a vegetable peeler to make ribbons down the length of each of the carrots and toss with the rice mixture. Divide between bowls, add the miso squares to the top, along with a few slices of radish, and sprinkle over extra chives to garnish.

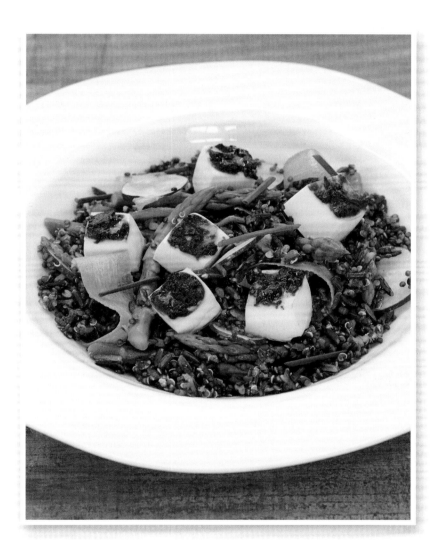

GREEN GAZPACHO WITH TOASTED TAMARI PUMPKIN SEEDS & FETA

This soup is best made in a powerful blender, such as a Vitamix or Nutribullet, though a food processor would be fine otherwise. If you prefer the texture creamier, add yoghurt in place of the water.

PREP TIME: 15 MINUTES
COOKING TIME: 4–6 MINUTES
MAKES: ABOUT 1.5 LITRES
SOUP / 6 SERVINGS

50g blanched hazelnuts
1 head of romaine lettuce
2 celery sticks, trimmed and
    roughly chopped
1 medium cucumber,
    roughly chopped
4 tbsp extra-virgin olive oil,
    or to taste
1 small (10g) bunch of mint,
    leaves picked
1 small (10g) bunch of
    coriander
2 cloves of garlic, peeled
1 green chilli, deseeded
3 tbsp apple cider vinegar
150ml water
sea salt and black pepper
100g feta cheese, crumbled,
    to serve

For the toasted pumpkin seeds
1 tsp olive oil
1 tsp tamari
50g pumpkin seeds

Toast the hazelnuts in a small non-stick frying pan over a medium-high heat for 2–3 minutes then allow to cool before placing in a blender or food processor with the lettuce, celery, cucumber, olive oil, mint, coriander, garlic and chilli. Blitz until smooth, then add the apple cider vinegar and the water and blitz again, thinning with more water if required.

Season with salt and pepper to taste, then place in the fridge to chill until you're ready to serve. This will keep for two days in an airtight container.

Heat the oil and tamari in the non-stick frying pan. Add the pumpkin seeds and toast for 2–3 minutes, stirring to coat them in the soy sauce and removing from the heat when they puff up. Drain on a piece of kitchen paper.

Divide the chilled gazpacho between bowls and top with the toasted pumpkin seeds and crumbled feta cheese.

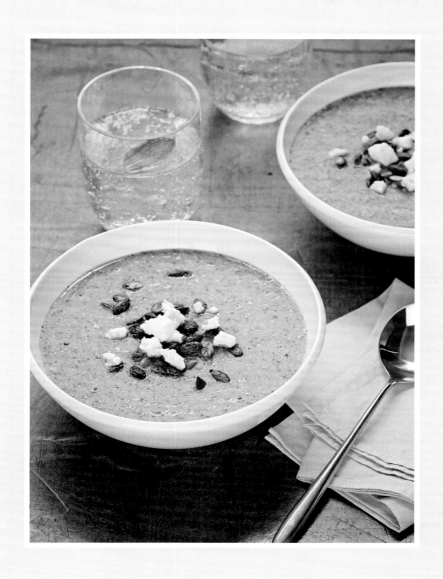

SPICE-CRUSTED CHICKEN WITH SWEET POTATO & TOMATO SALAD

Adding a spice rub to a simple chicken breast adds an extra impact of flavour to a relatively simple dish. Not only does bashing the chicken make for extra surface area to coat in the spice, it also speeds up the cooking time.

PREP TIME: 15 MINUTES
COOKING TIME:
1 HOUR 15–20 MINUTES
MAKES: 4 SERVINGS

4 x 125g skinless and boneless
　chicken breasts
2 x 350g sweet potatoes,
　unpeeled and scrubbed
250g plum tomatoes (about
　4 medium)
1 small (10g) bunch of flat-leaf
　parsley, leaves picked
30g creamed coconut
juice of ½ lime
pinch of sea salt
1 tbsp rapeseed oil

For the spice rub
1 tbsp ground allspice
1 tbsp dried thyme
½ tsp ground cinnamon
2 tsp sweet smoked paprika
½ tsp mild chilli powder
½ tsp black pepper
1 tsp sea salt
1 tsp coconut sugar

Preheat the oven to 200°C/180°C fan/gas 6.

Mix all the ingredients together for the spice rub. Take a chopping board and scatter half the mix across it. Lay the chickens on top and use a rolling pin to bash them, tenderising them and sealing the spices into the flesh while flattening them out to about 1cm thick. Place the chicken breasts in a plastic container and leave to marinate in the fridge while the sweet potatoes are cooking.

Prick the potatoes with a sharp knife and place on a baking tray in the oven. Cook for about 1 hour 15 minutes or until the flesh is soft and tender.

Meanwhile, chop the tomatoes into rough chunks and add to a medium bowl. Add the parsley leaves, grate in the coconut and squeeze in the lime juice, then season with a pinch of salt and set aside.

Shortly before the sweet potato is ready, heat a large griddle pan over a high heat. Drizzle the marinated chicken breasts with the rapeseed oil and fry for 3 minutes on each side or until cooked through and beautifully charred. If your griddle pan isn't large enough, simply cook the chicken in two batches. Cut the cooked chicken into strips.

Serve half a sweet potato per person with salad on top and the charred spicy chicken on the side.

WILD GARLIC PESTO
WITH RAW COURGETTI

This is a satisfying and simple dish to have up your sleeve on days
when you want a super quick lunch or if you get in late from work.
It requires no cooking and is absolutely delicious cold.

PREP TIME: 5 MINUTES
COOKING TIME: 10 MINUTES
MAKES: 2 SERVINGS

2 large courgettes, trimmed
1 large handful of wild garlic,
    stalks trimmed and leaves
    washed
50g Brazil nuts, or you can
    use unsalted almonds,
    cashews or pine nuts
1 handful of fresh spinach
    or watercress (optional)
about 100ml extra virgin
    olive oil
Parmesan, to serve (optional)
sea salt and black pepper

Use a spiraliser or vegetable peeler to create
thin spaghetti like strips or ribbons of courgette.
Split the strips between two serving bowls.

Place the wild garlic, nuts and spinach or
watercress, if using, in a small blender. Start to
blend and slowly add the oil in a constant dribble.
Don't add the oil all at once; you will need to
check the consistency as you go, so just add
a little at a time.

Once you have a semi-smooth paste, stir in some
seasoning and drizzle some over your courgetti.
Top with a few shavings of Parmesan if you like
and serve immediately.

Any extra pesto can be kept in a sealed jar in
the fridge for up to 1 week.

COLD BUCKWHEAT NOODLES WITH CRISPY GINGER & CHILLI PORK

I like to eat carbs at lunch rather than dinner and this exceedingly tasty combination is an excellent way of enjoying gluten-free soba noodles with crispy fried pork piled on top.

PREP TIME: 5 MINUTES
COOKING TIME: 15–20 MINUTES
MAKES: 4 SERVINGS

For the noodles
250g buckwheat (soba) noodles
3 tbsp sesame oil
1 tbsp black sesame seeds,
    plus 1 tbsp to serve

For the crispy pork
1 tbsp rapeseed oil
3cm knob of root ginger,
    peeled and grated
3 garlic cloves, peeled and
    finely chopped
2 red chillies, deseeded
    and finely chopped
4 spring onions, finely chopped
500g minced pork
1 tbsp coconut sugar
2 tbsp fish sauce (nam pla)
juice and finely grated zest
    of 1 lime
4 lime leaves, finely chopped
dried chilli flakes (optional)
sea salt

Cook the buckwheat noodles following the instructions on the packet. Once cooked and drained, toss lightly in the sesame oil and black sesame seeds and set aside to cool.

Heat the oil in a large sauté pan or frying pan (the pan needs to be wide or the mixture won't dry out properly) over a medium heat. Add the ginger, garlic and chillies and fry for 1 minute. Add the spring onions and continue to fry for a further minute. Tip in the pork and cook for another 2–3 minutes, breaking up the meat as it cooks to ensure that it does not form lumps. Sprinkle over the sugar, fish sauce, lime juice and zest, chopped lime leaves and a little salt.

Cook everything down until the juices have been absorbed and any liquid has evaporated so that the texture is almost crumb-like – this should take 10–15 minutes. Taste for spiciness: if you prefer a more fiery kick, add some dried chilli flakes. Divide the noodles between bowls and add the crispy pork to the top, along with an extra sprinkling of black sesame seeds.

COURGETTI WITH CLAMS, CHERRY TOMATOES & CHILLI

Spaghetti *alle vongole is* one of my all-time favourite meals. This version combines my newfound love of using a spiraliser with this Italian classic, making it a gluten-free and lighter way to enjoy this quintessential Italian dish.

PREP TIME: 10 MINUTES
COOKING TIME: 12–13 MINUTES
MAKES: 4 SERVINGS

2 large courgettes
1 tbsp rapeseed oil
1 red onion, peeled and
    finely chopped
2 tbsp capers, drained or
    rinsed (if in salt)
2 cloves of garlic, peeled
    and sliced
1 red chilli, deseeded and
    finely chopped
200g cherry tomatoes, halved
500g clams, scrubbed
500g mussels, scrubbed and
    de-bearded
1 small (10g) bunch of parsley,
    leaves picked and roughly
    chopped

Use a spiraliser to make spaghetti from the courgettes. (If you don't have a spiraliser, you can use a vegetable peeler to make long ribbons from the courgettes instead.) Set aside in a bowl.

Heat the rapeseed oil in a large sauté pan or saucepan (with a lid) over a medium-low heat. Add the red onion, capers, garlic and chilli and fry for 5 minutes. Add the cherry tomatoes and cook for a further 2 minutes.

Turn up the heat to high, add the clams and mussels and place the lid on the pan. Cook for 4–5 minutes, shaking the pan every once in a while. Remove the lid to check if the mussels and clams have opened, replacing the lid and cooking for a further minute or so if they need a bit longer.

If almost all of them are open, give them a stir and add the courgetti to the top of the pan, cooking the mixture for 1 minute with the lid off, then remove from the heat, toss everything around in the pan, sprinkle with the parsley and serve immediately. (Discard any mussels or clams that remain unopened.)

COCONUT & QUINOA
SEAFOOD SOUP

Laksa is one of my favourite comfort foods and this version has become a dinner-party staple, combining my beloved seafood with leafy greens and quinoa.

PREP TIME: 10 MINUTES
COOKING TIME: 35 MINUTES
MAKES: 2 SERVINGS

2 tbsp rapeseed oil
1 red onion, peeled and sliced
1 lemon grass stalk, peeled and
    bashed with the back of
    your knife
3 cloves of garlic, peeled
    and finely chopped
4cm knob of root ginger,
    peeled and thinly sliced
1 tsp turmeric
400ml coconut milk
400ml water, chicken
    or fish stock
100g red quinoa
6 raw king prawns, shells on
200g skinless white fish
    fillets, such as cod, haddock
    or monkfish
350g mussels, scrubbed
    and de-bearded
2 heads of bok choy,
    leaves separated

To serve
1 tbsp soy sauce or tamari
1 tbsp fish sauce (nam pla)
juice of 1 lime
1 small (10g) bunch of
    coriander, chopped
2 spring onions, sliced
    at an angle

Heat the oil in a medium saucepan (with a lid) over a medium heat. Once the oil is hot, add the red onion, lemon grass, garlic, ginger and turmeric. Fry for 10 minutes or until the onion is soft and the mixture fragrant, then add the coconut milk and water, chicken or fish stock. Bring to a simmer and cook for a further 15 minutes.

Strain the contents of the pan through a sieve into a bowl, then return the strained liquid to the pan (discarding what remains in the sieve) and bring back to a simmer. Add the quinoa and cook for 7 minutes, then tip in the prawns, white fish and mussels.

Bring the mixture back up to a simmer and place the bok choy on top of the liquid to steam. Pop the lid on the pan and give it a shake. Cook for a further 4 minutes or until the shells of the mussels have opened (discard any that don't) and the quinoa is cooked.

Remove from the heat. Add the soy sauce or tamari, along with the fish sauce and lime juice. Stir through, taste, adjusting with more soy or fish sauce if needed, and divide between bowls. Scatter with the coriander and chopped spring onions and serve immediately.

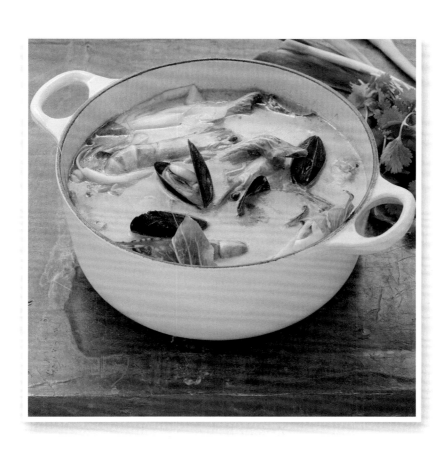

PAN-ROASTED SALMON, SHAVED BROCCOLI & GREEN BEANS WITH TAHINI-POPPY SEED DRESSING

This provides an excellent post-gym, protein-rich supper, which packs quite a colourful punch on the plate. A much-publicised superfood, turmeric is considered a highly effective anti-inflammatory, but it also makes a beautiful dress for this pretty green 'slaw'.

PREP TIME: 15 MINUTES
COOKING TIME: 12–15 MINUTES
MAKES: 4 SERVINGS

1 large head of broccoli
200g green beans, trimmed
2 tbsp olive oil
4 salmon fillets, skin
   on and pin-boned
sea salt and black pepper
1 lemon, cut into quarters,
   to serve

For the dressing
juice of ½ lemon
1½ tbsp tahini
2 tbsp extra-virgin olive oil
2 tbsp natural Greek yoghurt
   or coconut yoghurt
1 tbsp poppy seeds
¼ tsp turmeric

Using a mandolin or a sharp knife, finely slice the head of broccoli lengthways to get a mixture of florets and long strands of stalk. Add to a bowl with any leftover green crumbs.

Bring a small saucepan of salted water to the boil and add the green beans. Blanch for 2–3 minutes or until al dente, then drain in a colander and plunge into a bowl of cold water. Drain again and slice lengthways into thin strands before adding to the broccoli.

Make the dressing by mixing the lemon juice in a bowl with the tahini, olive oil, yoghurt, poppy seeds and turmeric. Whisk to combine, seasoning with salt and pepper to taste. Set aside.

Take a large sauté pan (with a lid), add the olive oil and place over a medium heat. Season the salmon fillets generously on both sides with salt and pepper. When the oil is hot, add the fillets, skin side down, and cook with the lid on for 10–12 minutes or until the skin is super-crisp and the flesh almost cooked through but still succulent. Remove from the pan, drain on kitchen paper and serve immediately with the salad, tossed in the dressing, and the lemon wedges.

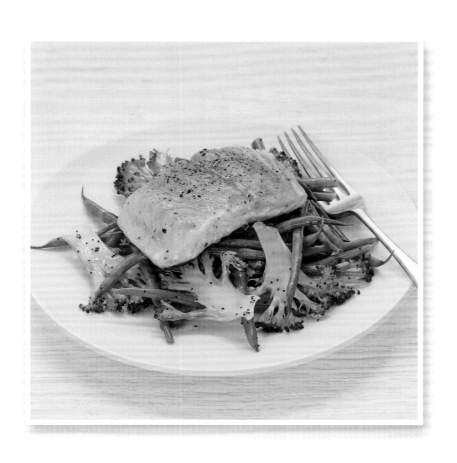

BAKED AUBERGINES WITH TOMATOES, FETA & THYME

This is one of my go-to store-cupboard-raid dinners –
effortlessly delicious and endlessly satisfying.

PREP TIME: 10 MINUTES
COOKING TIME: 40 MINUTES
MAKES: 2–4 SERVINGS

2 medium aubergines
2 tbsp olive oil
1 onion, peeled and
    finely chopped
3 cloves of garlic, peeled
    and sliced
1 x 400g tin of whole
    cherry tomatoes
2 tsp balsamic vinegar
8 sprigs of thyme
100g feta cheese
sea salt and black pepper

Preheat the oven to 180°C/160 fan/gas 4.

Cut the aubergines in half lengthways. Use a
spoon to scoop most of the flesh out, leaving about
1.5cm of flesh on the skin. Place on a baking tray,
drizzle with half the olive oil and a sprinkling of
salt and bake in the oven for 15–20 minutes while
you cook the sauce.

Heat the remaining oil in a medium saucepan
over a medium-low heat. Add the onion, garlic
and a pinch of salt and sweat for 5 minutes or until
the onion is translucent but not browned. Add the
tinned tomatoes and balsamic vinegar, season with
½ teaspoon each of salt and pepper, bring to a
simmer and cook for 15 minutes. Remove from the
heat and crush the tomatoes with a wooden spoon
if they haven't entirely broken down. Check the
seasoning, adjusting with more vinegar, salt or
pepper to taste.

Remove the aubergines from the oven and divide
the tomato sauce between them. Add 2 sprigs
of thyme to each one and then crumble the feta
over the top. Place back in the oven for a further
20 minutes or until soft and tender and the feta
has browned a little. Serve with a leafy salad on
the side as a light dinner.

MUSHROOM BUN BURGERS WITH HALLOUMI

This juicy burger is a twist on your classic brioche bun, using Portobello mushrooms as the bread component. You can make your own burger patties (the one below is very simply seasoned), or just buy them from your trusty butcher. I've cooked them on the grill here, but this recipe works really well on the barbecue otherwise.

PREP TIME: 5 MINUTES
COOKING TIME: 10–15 MINUTES
MAKES: 4 SERVINGS

400g lean minced beef
1 tsp sea salt
½ tsp ground black pepper
1–2 drops of Tabasco sauce
200g halloumi, sliced into 4
8 large Portobello mushrooms, stalks trimmed
3–4 tbsp rapeseed oil
4 round or iceberg lettuce leaves
1 beef tomato, sliced across into 4
1 small red onion, peeled and sliced into rounds
sriracha or other chilli sauce, to serve (optional)

Preheat your grill to medium-high and line a large baking tray with foil.

Mix the beef with the salt, pepper and Tabasco, massaging the seasoning into the meat. Form the mince into four burger patties and set aside.

Toss the halloumi slices and the Portobello mushrooms in the rapeseed oil and lay, spread apart, on the prepared baking tray. Place under the grill to cook for 8–10 minutes. After 4 minutes, turn them all over to cook on the other side and add the burger patties – they will take 3–4 minutes on each side. (The halloumi tends to take longer than the mushrooms, but it will depend on their size. You ultimately want the halloumi golden in places and the mushrooms soft but still holding their shape nicely.)

Once everything is cooked, assemble the buns. Place a mushroom on each plate, cap side down, and add a lettuce leaf, burger patty, tomato slice, onion rings and halloumi slice, then add another mushroom, rounded cap facing up. Repeat with the remaining ingredients to assemble all four buns. Serve with the chilli sauce, if desired.

VIETNAMESE CHICKEN MEATBALLS WITH MANGO, CHILLI & SPRING ONION SALSA

These chicken meatballs are massively versatile. As well as serving them for supper, I sometimes have them as a light lunch, tucked into lettuce leaves with plenty of the mango, chilli and spring onion salsa, or serve them up as finger food when I have friends over for drinks. If you're eating these as a more substantial meal, I'd suggest serving them on a bed of buckwheat noodles with shredded lettuce leaves tossed through for crunch.

PREP TIME: 10 MINUTES
COOKING TIME: 10 MINUTES
MAKES: 10–12 MEATBALLS /
2–4 SERVINGS

For the meatballs
1 red chilli, deseeded
3cm knob of root ginger,
    peeled and roughly chopped
1 large (20g) bunch of
    coriander, leaves and
    stalks separated
2 spring onions, roughly
    chopped
1 clove of garlic, peeled
grated zest and juice of 1 lime
2 tsp soy sauce or tamari
1 tsp fish sauce (nam pla)
1 tsp ground white pepper
1 x 270g skinless and boneless
    chicken breast or thigh,
    roughly chopped
2 tbsp olive oil
4 tbsp sesame seeds

Preheat the oven to 200°C/180°C fan/gas 6.

In a food processor, blend the red chilli, ginger and stalks from the bunch of the coriander with the spring onions, garlic, lime zest and 1½ tablespoons of the juice, the soy sauce or tamari, fish sauce and white pepper. Add the chicken and pulse a couple of times to form a rough mince. Roll the mixture into 10–12 bite-sized balls – you may need to wet your hands first if the mixture is sticky.

Pour the oil into a baking tray and place in the oven to heat up. Place the sesame seeds in a bowl and roll each chicken ball in them to coat. Remove the baking tray from the oven and add the meatballs, coating them in the oil. Place in the oven and bake for 10 minutes, shaking them in the pan after 5 minutes to ensure even browning.

Tip the peanuts, for serving, into a smaller baking tray or ovenproof dish and toast for 3–4 minutes

For the mango, chilli &
spring onion salsa
1 tbsp fish sauce (nam pla)
1 tbsp rice vinegar
lime juice (reserved from
    making the meatballs)
1 small mango, peeled,
    stoned and cubed
½–1 red chilli, sliced
2 spring onions, finely sliced
    into rounds

To serve
2 tbsp blanched, unsalted
    peanuts
1 Little Gem lettuce, leaves
    separated, or other lettuce
    leaves (optional)

in the oven at the same time as the meatballs, shaking the tray halfway through to prevent the nuts from burning.

In the meantime, make the salsa. In a bowl, mix the fish sauce with the vinegar and the remaining juice from the lime. Add the mango, chilli and the spring onions. Toss and check the seasoning, adjusting to taste, if needed, with more fish sauce or vinegar.

Serve the meatballs as suggested above, in lettuce leaves, with the salsa on the side and scattered with the roasted peanuts and coriander leaves.

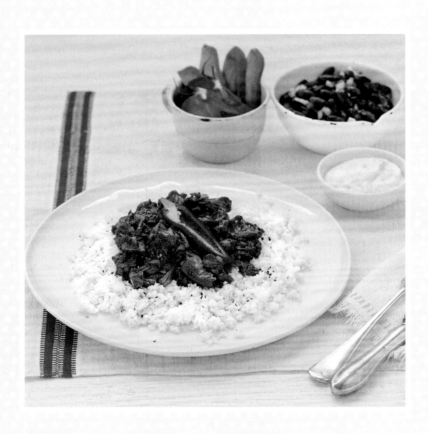

MELTING BEEF WITH CAULIFLOWER RICE

This is a bit of a Mexican-inspired feast, perfect for popping in the oven on a Sunday and letting it do the work for you. Cauliflower rice is a great healthy alternative to plain white rice, and it's even quicker to prepare, so do give it a go.

PREP TIME: 10 MINUTES
COOKING TIME: 4¼–4½ HOURS
MAKES: 4 SERVINGS

2 tbsp rapeseed oil
1 onion, peeled and finely chopped
2 cloves of garlic, peeled and finely chopped
750g boneless shin of beef, cut into 5cm chunks
160ml red wine
2 tbsp tomato purée
80ml water
160g tinned chopped tomatoes (about ½ x 400g tin)
1 red chilli, deseeded and finely chopped
1 level tsp sweet smoked paprika
1 dried chipotle chilli, left whole
sea salt and black pepper

For the cauliflower rice
½ large head of cauliflower
4 tbsp water
1 tbsp coconut oil

Preheat the oven to 150°C/130°C fan/gas 2.

Heat the oil in a flameproof, heavy-based casserole dish (with a tight-fitting lid) and add the finely chopped onion. Fry over a gentle heat for 10 minutes or until soft and transparent. Add the garlic and fry for the last 2 minutes. Tip the beef into the dish and brown lightly all over on a medium-high heat.

Pour in the red wine, bring to a simmer and deglaze the casserole dish, scraping any caramelised bits of meat or onion from the bottom of the dish. In a small bowl, mix the tomato purée with the water and add to the beef, along with the chopped tomatoes, chilli, paprika, chipotle and ½ teaspoon each of salt and pepper.

Bring all the ingredients to a simmer, cover with the lid and cook for about 5 minutes on the top of the stove. Dampen a piece of greaseproof paper with water and lay over the meat mixture in the casserole dish.

Put the lid back on the dish, place in the oven and cook for 4–4¼ hours. (The timing may vary according to your oven.) Check after a couple of

Recipe continues overleaf

hours and make sure that the meat is not drying out. You don't want too much liquid, but you do need the meat to retain its moist succulence. Add a little more water or wine if it seems to be drying out too much, and continue cooking until the meat is meltingly tender. Season with extra salt and pepper to taste when the meat is fully cooked.

Shortly before the beef is cooked, make the cauliflower rice. Pulse the cauliflower in a food processor or grate by hand into pieces roughly resembling the size and shape of grains of rice. Put the water and coconut oil in a large saucepan (with a tight-fitting lid) and bring to the boil. Add the cauliflower, cover with the lid and return the pan to a high heat for about 60 seconds.

Before serving, remove the beef from the casserole dish and shred with two forks, mixing in some or all of juices that remain in the dish. Divide the rice between plates and top with the beef, seasoning with salt and pepper to taste. This would be delicious served with red kidney beans (warmed through in a pan before serving, if using tinned), sliced beef tomatoes, avocado wedges and sour cream, if you like.

SEARED BEEF WITH CHIMICHURRI & SWEET POTATO CHIPS

This zippy Argentine sauce goes brilliantly with beef and, paired
with these sweet potato chips, makes for a dish that's as much
a joy on the plate as it is on the palate.

PREP TIME: 10 MINUTES
COOKING TIME: 45 MINUTES
MAKES: 4 SERVINGS

3 medium-sized sweet
    potatoes, unpeeled
    and scrubbed
4 tbsp rapeseed oil
4 fillet steaks (about 170g each),
    removed from the fridge
    30 minutes before cooking
sea salt and black pepper

For the chimichurri
100ml red wine vinegar
1 small (10g) bunch of oregano,
    very finely chopped
1 small (10g) bunch of parsley,
    very finely chopped
3 cloves of garlic, peeled and
    finely sliced or chopped
1 red chilli, deseeded and
    finely chopped
¼ red onion, peeled and
    finely chopped
2 tbsp extra-virgin olive oil

Preheat the oven to 200°C/180°C fan/gas 6 and
line a large baking tray with foil.

Cut the sweet potatoes into 1cm-wide chips and
place in the prepared baking tray. Toss the chips
in half the rapeseed oil, sprinkle with plenty of sea
salt and bake in the oven, spread well apart (this
will help them get crispy), for 30–40 minutes,
turning them over halfway through, or until
golden brown.

In the meantime, make the chimichurri. Mix all
the ingredients together in a small bowl, seasoning
with a generous pinch of salt, and set aside.

Heat the remaining rapeseed oil in a large frying
pan over a medium-high heat. If there is enough
room in the pan for all the fillets, cook together;
if not, cook in two batches to avoid crowding the
pan. Season the fillets on both sides with plenty
of salt and pepper. Once the pan is very hot, add
the fillets and cook for 2½–3½ minutes per side for
rare, or 3½–4½ minutes per side for medium rare.
Set aside to rest for 2 minutes, before slicing into
1cm slices – or serve whole, if you prefer.

Serve the fillets with the chimichurri drizzled
on top and the sweet potato chips on the side.

OVERNIGHT CHIA & ALMOND MILK PUDDING

This chia pudding is a bit of a revelation. The seeds plump up as they soak in the almond milk, creating an intriguing texture that works really well as dessert or a protein-packed breakfast.

PREP TIME: 2 MINUTES
CHILLING TIME: 2–3 HOURS
OR OVERNIGHT
MAKES: 6 SERVINGS

80g chia seeds
500ml almond milk
1 tbsp maple syrup

To serve
1–2 tbsp natural yoghurt
   or coconut yoghurt
1–2 tbsp berries, passion fruit
   or sliced mango or bananas

Measure the chia seeds into a small glass bowl or plastic container with the almond milk and maple syrup. Stir well to ensure that the chia seeds are completely covered. Cover with cling film or the plastic lid and chill in the fridge for a minimum of 2–3 hours, or preferably overnight to be ready for breakfast.

When you are ready to serve, give the mixture a really good stir. If you find it too stiff and set, you can loosen it with a little extra almond milk. Place a generous spoonful into a bowl, add some yoghurt to the top and your choice of berries or other fruit.

HOMEMADE PINK FRO-YO

You can add a touch of maple syrup if you don't find this recipe sweet enough, but I prefer to keep it au naturel. The mixture can also be frozen into ice-lolly moulds and eaten as ice lollies .(See picture on page 169).

(See picture on page 169)

PREP TIME: 10 MINUTES
FREEZING TIME: 2–3 HOURS
MAKES: 600G FROZEN
YOGHURT / 6 SERVINGS

4–6 ripe bananas
  (about 250g peeled flesh)
175g frozen mixed summer
  berries
250g natural Greek yoghurt
  or coconut yoghurt

For the toppings (optional)
1 tbsp coconut chips
1 tbsp goji berries
1 tbsp chopped pistachio
  kernels

Peel the bananas, chop into chunks and place in an airtight plastic container with a lid. Seal and pop in the freezer for 2–3 hours to freeze.

Once frozen, remove from the freezer and place in a food processor with the frozen berries and yoghurt. Blend to a soft-serve texture of frozen yoghurt. Serve immediately with or without a few sprinkles of one of the suggested toppings.

SUPERSEED CRACKERS WITH BLACK OLIVE TAPENADE

These crispy crackers make excellent little post-gym pick-me-ups. Keep a stash in your handbag for an instant energy boost. They go brilliantly with this tasty tapenade too.

PREP TIME: 15 MINUTES
COOKING TIME: 1 HOUR
RESTING TIME: 10–15 MINUTES
MAKES: ABOUT 40 CRACKERS

60g sunflower seeds
65g pumpkin seeds
40g sesame seeds
35g ground flaxseed
45g chia seeds
200ml water
1 tsp sea salt

For the tapenade
200g pitted black olives
    (Kalamata are best)
3 tbsp capers, rinsed and
    drained
2 cloves of garlic, peeled
juice of ½ lemon
3 tbsp extra-virgin olive oil
2–3 tinned anchovies (optional)

Preheat the oven to 170°C/150°C fan/gas 3.

Measure the seeds into a medium-large bowl and pour the water over the top. Leave to rest for 10–15 minutes, allowing the chia seeds to plump up and get sticky.

Take two large sheets of baking parchment, spread the seed mixture across one of the pieces and sprinkle the sea salt over the top. Place the second piece of baking parchment on top and use a rolling pin to evenly roll out the mixture to a rectangle about 4mm-thick. Lay the whole thing on a large baking tray and bake in the oven for 30 minutes. (If you have a baking sheet – one that's completely flat and without a 'lip' – you could instead line it with baking parchment, add the seed mixture and a second sheet of paper and roll out the mixture while it's on the baking sheet.)

After 30 minutes, remove from the oven, taking off the top piece of baking parchment, and use a sharp knife to make light indentations marking out the size and shape of your crackers – I tend to go for 4cm squares.

Return to the oven to bake for a further 30 minutes or until the crackers are totally crisp. Remove from the oven and break into the cracker shapes. Leave to cool on a wire rack and store in an airtight container for up to one week.

In the meantime, make the tapenade. In a food processor, blend all the ingredients together to a paste. Add extra oil to make the consistency thinner, if you wish. Serve with the seedy crackers.

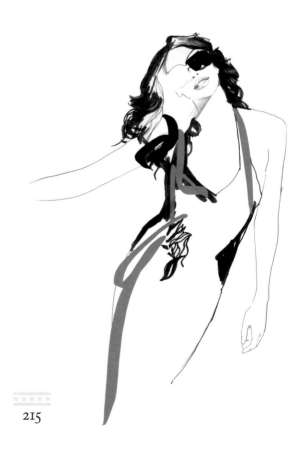

LEMONY ROAST CHICKEN

Is there anything more appealing than a roast chicken? My version combines a north African perennial, the preserved lemon, which I like to keep in my store cupboard. It's delicious served with fresh green vegetables, such as kale steamed with a spritz of lemon or a large green salad.

PREP TIME: 10 MINUTES
COOKING TIME: 1¼–1½ HOURS
MAKES: 4 SERVINGS

30g butter, softened
4 preserved lemons, roughly
  chopped
1 small (10g) bunch of thyme,
  leaves stripped
6 cloves of garlic, peeled
4 red onions, peeled and cut
  into quarters
1 whole chicken (about 1.4 kg)
1 lemon, halved
250ml white wine
100ml water
1 tbsp olive oil
sea salt and black pepper

Preheat the oven to 200°C/180°C fan/gas 6.

Place the butter, preserved lemons, thyme leaves, garlic and some salt and pepper in a food processor and blend until smooth. Put the onions in a roasting tin and place the chicken on top.

With your fingers, gently loosen the skin above the breast of the chicken, keeping the skin intact but creating enough space to slip the butter mixture right the way through. Insert the thyme stalks into the cavity of the chicken, along with the lemon halves. Add the white wine to the roasting tin, along with the water. Pat the chicken skin dry with kitchen paper and spread with the olive oil. Place in the oven and cook for 1¼–1½ hours, reducing the oven temperature to 190°C/170°C fan/gas 5 after the first 20 minutes.

When the chicken is ready – it should be brown and crispy on top and the juices should run clear when pierced with a skewer in the thickest part of the meat – remove from the oven. Leave the chicken on a board to rest before carving and drizzling with the juices from the tin.

STEPHEN'S ROAST POTATOES

When we are having a roast Stephen will always prepare the potatoes –
these are so full of flavour and really delicious! They go perfectly with
the Lemony Roast Chicken opposite.

PREP TIME: 10 MINUTES
COOKING TIME: 1 HOUR
MAKES: 4 SERVINGS

4 large Maris Piper potatoes,
   peeled and cut into chunks
2–3 tbsp olive oil
4 sprigs of rosemary
4 cloves of garlic, unpeeled
sea salt and black pepper

Preheat the oven to 200°C/180°C fan/gas 6.

Place the potatoes in a large saucepan, cover with cold salted water and bring to the boil. Once it has come to the boil, lower the heat and simmer for 15 minutes or until slightly tender.

While the potatoes are cooking, put the oil in a roasting tin and place in the oven to heat. Drain the potatoes in a colander and let the steam escape, tossing them around in the colander to break up the outside a bit. While still hot, carefully place the potatoes, rosemary and garlic cloves in the hot oil, season with plenty of salt and place in the oven for 45 minutes, tossing every 15 minutes or so to evenly brown them.

SLOW-ROAST PORK BELLY WITH RED CABBAGE & CRANBERRIES

Pork belly is one of my favourite cuts to roast. It's excellent value, juicy and succulent – and who doesn't love a bit of crispy crackling? The red cabbage and mashed potato complements it so well, too.

PREP TIME: 25 MINUTES
COOKING TIME: 3–3½ HOURS
MAKES: 4 SERVINGS

1 tsp fennel seeds
1–1.2kg boneless pork belly, skin well scored (ask your butcher to do this)
6 banana shallots, peeled and halved
2 eating apples, unpeeled, cored and quartered
250ml white wine
150ml chicken stock
sea salt and black pepper

For the red cabbage
1 tbsp butter
½ head of red cabbage, core removed and leaves finely shredded lengthways
50ml apple cider vinegar
2 tbsp agave syrup
75g frozen cranberries

For the mashed potato
600g King Edward potatoes, peeled and cut into chunks
4 tbsp butter

Preheat the oven to 230°C/210°C fan/gas 8.

Toast the fennel seeds in a dry pan for 2–3 minutes, then place in a mortar with 1½ teaspoons of sea salt and 1 teaspoon of freshly ground black pepper. Grind to a rough powder with the pestle.

Remove the pork belly from its packaging, pat the skin dry with kitchen paper if necessary (this helps make good crackling) and rub all over with the fennel seasoning. Take particular care rubbing it well into the scored skin. Place in a roasting tin and cook in the oven for about 1 hour or until the skin has turned golden brown and crackled. Remove from the oven and lower the temperature to 130°C/110°C fan/gas mark ½. Drain the fat from the roasting tin and discard.

Place the shallots and apples in the roasting tin with the pork belly. Add the wine and stock to the base of the tin (don't pour it over the pork belly skin – you want to keep that as dry as possible for the crackling). Cook for a further 2–2½ hours.

After the pork has been cooking for about 1¾ hours, place the potatoes in a large saucepan, cover with boiling water and add a pinch of salt. Cover with a lid and simmer for 20–25 minutes, until completely tender and soft. Drain the potatoes in a colander and transfer back to the saucepan. Use a potato masher or whisk to break up the potatoes and add the butter and some more salt and pepper.

Shortly before the pork is ready, make the red cabbage. Take a large sauté pan (with a lid) and set over a medium heat. Add the butter and melt until it starts to bubble, then tip in the cabbage. Cook for 2 minutes, then add the apple cider vinegar and agave syrup, tossing them with the cabbage. Add the frozen cranberries and season with ½ teaspoon of salt and a few grinds of pepper.

Place the lid on the pan and lower the heat to medium-low. Cook for 8–10 minutes, checking on it every so often. When the cabbage has softened, check the seasoning and adjust with more syrup or vinegar if you want it sharper or sweeter.

When the pork is done, it should feel very tender when prodded with a fork. Remove the pork, apples and shallots from the tin and leave to rest on a carving board in a warm place, covered with foil, while you make the gravy.

Pour the juices from the pan into a jug, let settle and then skim off the fat. Discard the fat, return the juices to a small saucepan and simmer to achieve a thicker consistency. Check seasoning.

Serve chunks of crackling with the pork, mash, some red cabbage and a drizzle of the gravy.

DAMSON RIPPLE ROULADE

I like to use my mum's homemade damson purée for this recipe, as it makes such a wonderful tangy contrast with the meringue and cream, but a shop-bought summer berry compote would work equally well otherwise. The recipe makes around 400g of purée; you only need half (about 200g) for this dish, but the rest will keep in the fridge for up to a week and is delicious stirred into yoghurt or spread on toast. The meringue roulade can be made up to a day ahead and stored in the fridge; it freezes well too.

PREP TIME: 15 MINUTES
COOKING TIME: 40 MINUTES
MAKES: 8 SERVINGS

rapeseed oil, for oiling
5 egg whites
275g caster sugar
50g flaked almonds (optional)
300ml double cream, or 150ml
    mascarpone mixed with
    150ml crème fraîche

For the damson purée
(makes 400g)
500g damsons
200ml water
125g caster sugar

To make the damson purée, place the damsons and water in a large saucepan, bring to the boil and then lower the heat and let simmer for 15 minutes or until tender. When they are cooked, pour the damsons into a sieve placed over a bowl and use a wooden spoon to push the damson flesh through the sieve, leaving the skins and stones behind. Stir in the sugar and taste, adding more sugar if necessary. Allow to cool and store in a clean, lidded jar in the fridge.

When you are ready to make the roulade, preheat the oven to 200°C/180°C fan/gas 6, then line the base of a 23cm x 33cm Swiss roll tin with baking parchment and grease with a little rapeseed oil.

Using an electric hand mixer, whisk the egg whites in a clean, dry bowl until they stand in stiff peaks, then slowly add the sugar and whisk at a high speed until glossy.

Spoon the mixture into the prepared tin, spreading it out evenly, and sprinkle over the almonds, if using. Place in the oven to cook for 8 minutes, then turn down the heat to 160°C/140°C fan/gas 2½ and cook for another 15 minutes or until the meringue is lightly browned and crisp to touch.

Remove from the oven and immediately turn out, nut side down if using the nuts, onto a piece of baking parchment. Peel the paper from the bottom of the meringue and leave to cool for 10 minutes.

Whip the cream, if using, into stiff peaks then spread this (or the mixture of mascarpone and crème fraîche) all over the meringue. Using about half the damson purée, trail over the cream in lines or blobs.

With one of the long sides facing you, roll the roulade tightly, using the paper to help you, and chill in the fridge until ready to serve.

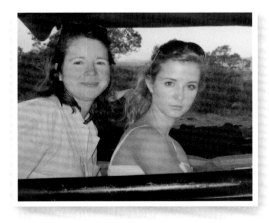

BANANA & BRAN MUFFINS WITH ROASTED RHUBARB JAM

A healthier take on this ever-popular little cake, these bran and banana muffins are a favourite in my family for snacking on at any time of day. Serving them with the rhubarb turns them into more of a dessert or a breakfast treat.

PREP TIME: 10 MINUTES
COOKING TIME:
35–40 MINUTES
MAKES: 6 MUFFINS

2 tbsp butter, melted and
    slightly cooled, plus extra
    for greasing if needed
60g organic wheat bran
150g plain flour
½ tsp baking powder
½ tsp bicarbonate of soda
80g panela sugar, plus 1–2 tbsp
    extra for sprinkling
½ tsp sea salt
120ml natural yoghurt
120ml water
1 medium egg
1 medium banana (about
    90g peeled flesh), mashed
1 tbsp agave syrup
100g dried cranberries
    (optional)

For the roasted rhubarb jam
200g rhubarb (about 4 sticks),
    trimmed and cut into
    5cm pieces
50ml maple syrup

Preheat the oven to 170°C/150°C fan/gas 3 and line a six-cup muffin tin with paper cases or grease each hole with butter.

Spread the bran out on a baking tray and place in the oven to toast for about 10 minutes, shaking the tray after 5 minutes to prevent the bran from burning. Remove from the oven and set aside, then turn the oven temperature up to 200°C/180°C fan/gas 6.

Sift the flour, baking powder and bicarbonate of soda into a bowl. Stir in the toasted bran with the sugar and salt. In a separate large bowl, mix together the yoghurt, water, egg, mashed banana, melted butter and agave syrup, whisking lightly to combine.

Tip the dry ingredients, including half the cranberries if you are using them, onto the liquid mixture and mix very lightly. The consistency should be that of a thick batter.

Spoon the batter into the prepared muffin tin, being sure that they are actually full or even slightly over-full. If you are using the dried cranberries, then scatter over the remaining berries as evenly as you can, pushing them into the top of each muffin.

Place in the oven to bake for about 25 minutes or until well risen and golden and a skewer inserted into one of the muffins comes out clean.

While the muffins are baking, toss the rhubarb in the maple syrup and place in a small baking dish. Place in the oven to bake for 20 minutes or until tender but not mushy. Remove from the oven and mash it up with a fork to give it a rough texture.

As soon as you remove the muffins from the oven, sprinkle with the extra panela sugar. Serve alongside some of the roasted rhubarb.

NUTTY BUTTER & SEED COOKIES

These deliciously nutty cookies are packed with goodness, the ideal snack for enjoying with a hot drink or to carry around in your handbag if you're out and about. They keep well in a cookie jar or airtight container for at least a week – if you can resist them!

PREP TIME: 10 MINUTES
COOKING TIME:
30–35 MINUTES
MAKES: 10 COOKIES

55g coconut oil
60ml maple syrup
75g unsweetened almond
    butter
½ tsp sea salt
7 soft prunes or dates, pitted
    and very finely chopped
100g porridge oats
    (I use gluten-free ones)
100g mixed seeds (mix
    of sunflower, pumpkin,
    golden linseed, hemp
    and sesame seeds)
70g ground almonds
1 medium egg

Preheat the oven to 180°C/160°C fan/gas 4 and line a large baking tray with baking parchment.

Place the coconut oil in a small saucepan with the maple syrup, almond butter, salt and prunes or dates and heat gently, stirring until all the ingredients are thoroughly mixed together. Add the oats to a bowl with the mixed seeds, ground almonds and egg, and stir to combine. Tip the contents of the pan into the bowl and mix everything together.

Form the cookie mixture into ten cookies, wetting your hands lightly and moulding each cookie in the palm of your hand. Lay them out on the prepared baking tray – they don't spread out as they bake, so you can place them just 2cm apart.

Place in the oven to bake for 30–35 minutes or until crispy and golden on the outside and still a bit chewy in the middle. Place on a wire rack to cool before storing.

LEMON POLENTA & ALMOND CAKE

One of my favourite cakes of all time, it works both as a snack
or as a dessert, served with a dollop of crème fraîche.

PREP TIME: 10 MINUTES
COOKING TIME:
55–60 MINUTES
MAKES: 8 SERVINGS

200g butter, softened,
    plus extra for greasing
225g caster sugar
½ tsp vanilla extract
pinch of sea salt
finely grated zest and juice
    of 2 unwaxed lemons
3 eggs, lightly beaten
200g ground almonds
150g quick-cook polenta
1 heaped tsp baking powder
3 tbsp agave syrup
3 tbsp nibbed pistachios
100g crème fraîche, to serve
    (optional)

Preheat the oven to 150°C/130°C fan/gas 2,
then grease the base of a 20cm-diameter
springform cake tin with butter and line
with baking parchment.

Cream the butter with the caster sugar, vanilla
extract and salt until light and fluffy. (You can do
this by hand or in a food mixer.) Add the lemon
zest and beat again to incorporate before adding
the eggs one by one and mixing until all the
ingredients are thoroughly combined.

In a separate bowl, mix the ground almonds
with the polenta and baking powder. Add the
dry ingredients to the creamed mixture and fold
in until evenly incorporated before pouring into
the prepared cake tin. Use a spatula to even out
the surface and place in the centre of the oven.

Bake for 55–60 minutes or until a skewer inserted
in the centre comes out clean. Leave to cool in the
tin for 10 minutes while you mix the lemon juice
with the agave syrup. Whisk until the mixture is
well combined then pour over the cake evenly.
Scatter the pistachios on top.

Serve as the cake as it is or with crème fraîche,
if you fancy. As this is so moist, this keeps well
for up to 2–3 days in an airtight container.

COCONUT, CARDAMOM & BITTER CHOCOLATE TRUFFLES

I come from a family of chocolatiers, so I have to credit them
for my love of very dark chocolate. These dairy-free truffles
are just as creamy as their lactic counterparts.

PREP TIME: 15 MINUTES
COOKING TIME: 5 MINUTES
SETTING TIME: 1–2 HOURS
MAKES: ABOUT 20 TRUFFLES

150g coconut cream
pinch of sea salt
200g dark chocolate
    (80% cocoa solids),
    finely chopped
¼ tsp ground cardamom
    (optional)

For the toppings
1 tbsp raw cacao powder
1 tbsp freeze-dried
    raspberry powder
1 tbsp desiccated coconut

Place the coconut cream, salt and chocolate in a
heatproof bowl set over a pan of gently simmering
water. (The bottom of the bowl should not touch
the water.)

Leave the chocolate to melt (stirring only
occasionally) before pouring into a 500ml plastic
container and placing in the fridge to set for
1–2 hours.

Once the chocolate has set, scoop into teaspoon-
sized balls and roll in the three different toppings
(or roll in 3 tablespoons of just one of the
toppings). Place in a separate plastic container
and store in the fridge until eating (they will keep
for 2–3 days).

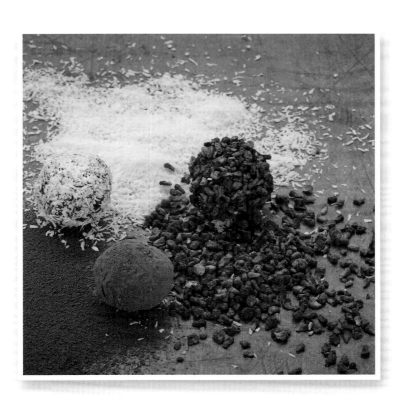

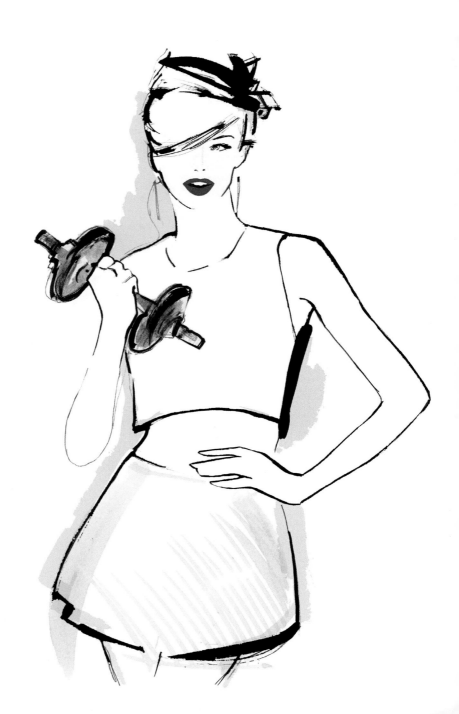

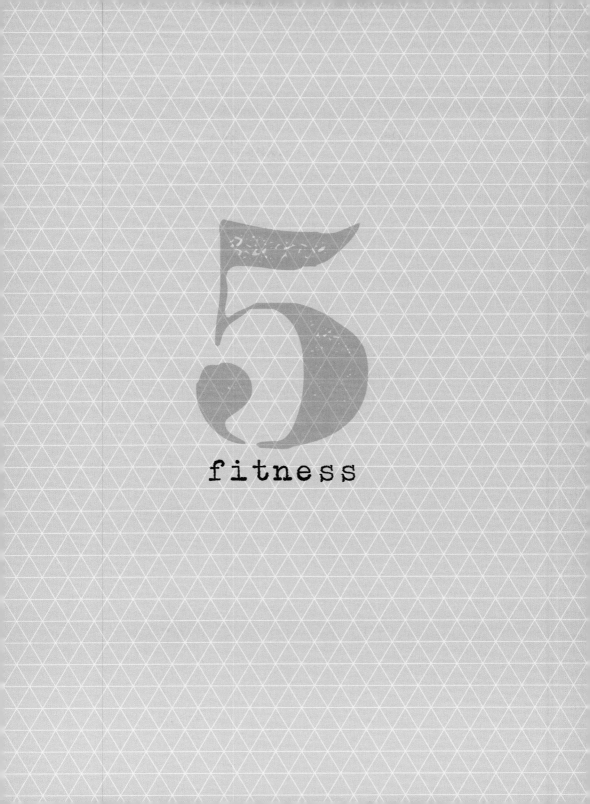

5

fitness

Fitness is a relatively new discovery for me. I always hated sport at school: lacrosse and hockey just meant bruises; cross-country running made me feel as though I couldn't breathe; and swimming frightened me. In the sixth form, we could choose our sport, so I opted for yoga and just went to sleep on my mat.

Complacency was a big part of it – I have always been naturally slim, so, as a teenager, I couldn't really see the point of exercise – but it wasn't the whole story. My dyspraxia means that I'm quite uncoordinated and that put me off going to classes. When I was first living in London, my friend started going to an aerobics class, but I was so hideously embarrassed about the thought of being out of sync and not keeping up that I refused to go with her. I walked out of the first proper yoga class I tried.

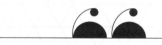

Exercise is not just about looking better; being fit makes you feel so much better too

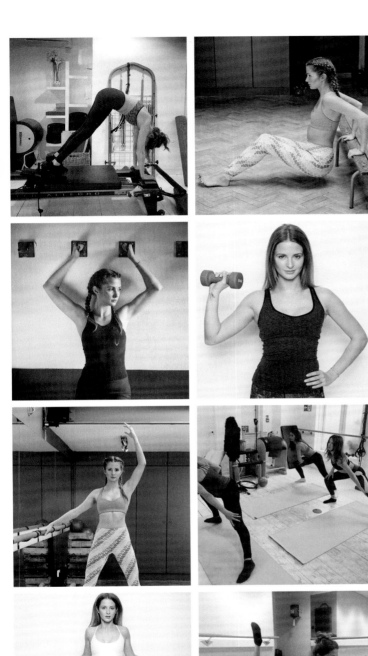
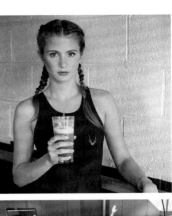
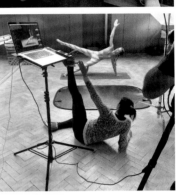
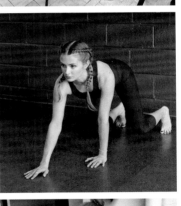
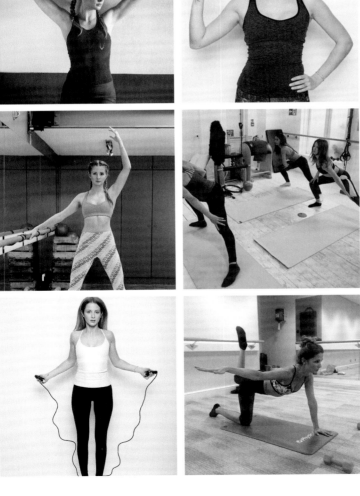
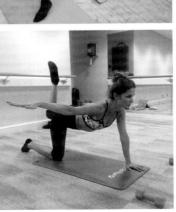
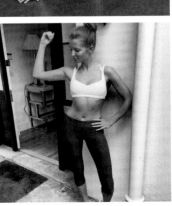

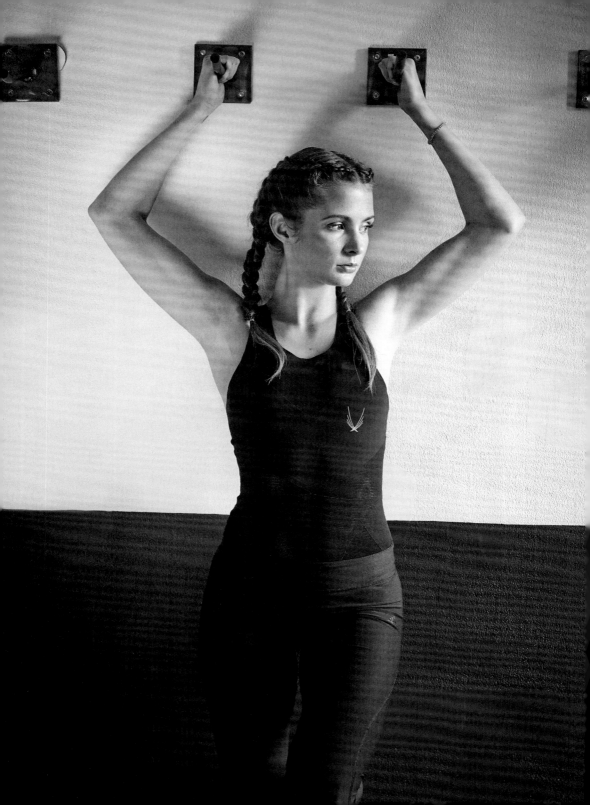

Everything changed when I started seeing Stephen's trainer a few months before our wedding. I had noticed that I was developing a muffin top and an extra chin and, of course, I wanted to look my best in my dress. I was feeling pretty focused (there's nothing like a bit of vanity to spur you on), but when I started it certainly wasn't love at first sight! I met the trainer in this real sweat and sawdust gym and he put me through a routine than involved battle ropes (huge ropes anchored to a wall that work every muscle group simultaneously), sandbags, a rowing machine, burpees and kettlebell weights. I was horrified by how hard it was and could scarcely walk for days.

It took time to see any improvement, but after a few months of pretty intensive training, I noticed that I was getting leaner. First, my arms, shoulders and legs started to feel more solid and then my mid-section began to firm up too. I'd be lying if I said it was easy – there were times when I left the gym feeling physically sick, and there are still mornings when I'd much rather stay in bed than turn up for a training session – but I like the results. I like seeing definition in my arms, legs and stomach. But exercise is not just about looking better; I've found that being fit makes me feel better too. Training is therapy for the brain. It doesn't matter how stressful life is, when I start a workout, I have to focus, so by the time I'm done, I'm physically exhausted but mentally alert and buzzing with fresh ideas. Improving at the gym also gives me a sense of achievement – the knowledge that my body is strong enables me to believe in myself a bit more.

I've been lucky enough to have worked with some wonderful trainers and I've also got over my self-consciousness about classes (everybody's concentrating too hard to watch anyone else), which means that I've discovered some brilliant ways to train like Ballet Barre and boxing. This chapter is all about passing on my passion and sharing some of the things I've been taught.

MOTIVATION

Fitness is a lifelong, personal journey. There is no sense in comparing yourself to others, because it's not about being better than other people; it's about being better than you used to be. Getting started can be hard and as exercising when you're unfit is tough, it can be even harder to keep going, but while persistence and consistency are essential, they really do pay off. Here are a few things that helped me:

 # FIND SOMETHING YOU ENJOY. Working out won't become part of your life if you hate the sessions. Look for something that will stimulate and challenge you. I really like variety so I do lots of different classes, but I'm always keen to work on my core muscles.

 # INVEST IN SOME NICE KIT. When I started, my gym kit consisted of a pair of shapeless leggings, a bobbly T-shirt and some old tennis shoes, which did nothing for my self-confidence. Treat yourself to something that makes you feel good. Obviously, it needs to fit well, provide enough support and absorb sweat, but there are lots of different styles around, so you can choose a shape to flatter your figure. I like to wear leggings (I have lots of pairs in a variety of lengths and ranging in colour from plain black to brightly patterned) and a cropped top with a built-in bra. Crop tops are great for Pilates because they enable you – and your teacher – to see your core muscles and see if they are switched on. I like to co-ordinate my tops with my trainers. (Seek specialist advice when choosing trainers – what you need will depend on the sport, you can get so many types now.)

 # TRAIN WITH A FRIEND. My Saturday morning ritual is a gym class with my girlfriends, followed by brunch.

SET A GOAL. I had my wedding to focus on, but it could be a birthday party or a holiday.

BE REALISTIC. If you tell yourself that you're going to train seven days a week, then you're setting yourself up to fail (and do yourself an injury). Work out a programme that's sustainable. I train four to five times a week because keeping really fit has become part of my job, but three times a week should be enough to make a visible difference. Anything is definitely better than nothing, though.

MONITOR YOUR PROGRESS. Taking a picture of yourself in your underwear each week will help you to see changes.

STRETCH. You must warm up at the start of a session, and stretch properly at the end to lengthen your muscles and improve flexibility.

a note on body types

Regular training can turn fat into lean muscle, leaving you slimmer and firmer, but it can't work magic. I have quite a flat chest and no amount of work in the gym is going to change that. You will save yourself a lot of disappointment by identifying your basic body type and learning to love its characteristics. There are three basic body types:

★ ECTOMORPHS – characterised by long, thin limbs and light muscle
★ ENDOMORPHS – characterised by rounder limbs that gain muscle easily but are prone to store fat
★ MESMOMORPHS – characterised by strong, muscular limbs

★ ★ ★ ★ ★

CLASSES

Now that I've got over my embarrassment, I try to go to several different classes every week. I aim for two cardio workouts, two weight sessions, a Pilates or Ballet Barre class and one yoga session each week. The ones I've included here are my personal favourites, but there are many others to choose from. The free app Mindbody Connect is a brilliant tool for helping you find a class. Just type in your postcode, select the class you're looking for and it will tell you where the nearest one is. It has a wellness directory too – great for hunting down a local acupuncturist, chiropractor or spa.

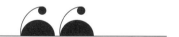

If you feel nervous about attending classes on your own, ask a friend to go with you – this will give you motivation and confidence

PAOLA'S BODYBARRE (PBB)

Ballet barre is a combination of ballet and Pilates, which involve both a barre and a floor mat. I like it because the focus is on toning the stomach and core and it gets into those really deep, hard-to-reach muscles. I'm all about seeing results and after six months of doing these classes, I noticed that my bum had lifted. It's improved my co-ordination, posture and flexibility too – now, when I'm warmed up, I can do a standing leg raise with both hands on the floor.

I asked the wonderful Paola Di Lanzo of Paola's BodyBarre to devise six simple, at-home exercises that you can do using the back of a chair as a barre – try them and get hooked!

note

All these exercises are done with a Pilates breath – i.e. inhaling through your nose to prepare and exhaling through your mouth with pursed lips as you go into the exertion phase of the exercise. Make sure that you 'centre', drawing your navel towards the spine, with every exhalation.

PBB DANCER'S STRETCH

This full-body stretch is a great way of opening the hips and shoulders and is a useful one to do in between any exercise that uses the quads, such as the plié (see page 240). It also strengthens the spine and releases tension in the ankle and foot, helping to prevent injury.

#1

Stand square on to – and a full arm's distance away from – the barre/chair back. With your right hand resting on the barre/chair, bend your left leg back and hold onto the inside of your foot with your left hand.

#2

Inhale then exhale as you extend the left side of your body, sending your left foot up towards the ceiling. Make sure that you are pushing your foot into your hand. Extend the back of your neck as you gaze forwards. Hold the pose for 10–20 seconds.

#3

Repeat on the other side.

#4

To improve your balance, try the exercise with your right arm extended in front of you rather than resting on the barre/chair back, then repeat on the other side with your left arm extended in front of you.

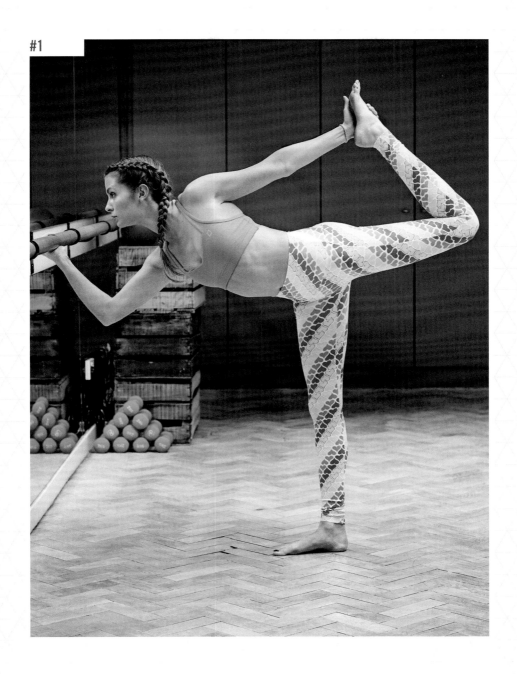

PBB GRAND PLIÉ IN SECOND POSITION ON DEMI POINTE

This exercise – stretching from a deep knee bend (grand plié) on the balls of your feet (demi pointe) – is good for toning your thighs, glutes and calves.

#1

Standing side on to the barre/chair back and with your right hand placed lightly on it, step out into second position (feet more than a shoulder width apart), raising your heels off the floor to demi pointe (the balls of your feet). Be sure to keep your feet and knees turned out, each knee tracking the big toe.

#2

Place your left arm in first position (at thigh level with your hand curving in).

#3

Bend your knees so your thighs are parallel, or almost parallel, with the floor and keep your pelvis in neutral (without tipping it up or down).

#4

As you rise up, straightening your legs, draw your inner thighs in, pull your knees up and squeeze your glutes. Your free arm should rise to fifth position (above your head with your hand curving in) as you lift, and lower back down to first position as you bend your knees again.

#5

Repeat 15–20 times, finishing with 20 small, downward pulses.

#6

Repeat on the other side.

#7

As an optional extra to work the shoulders and biceps, repeat the exercise on each side holding a 1–1.5kg weight in your free hand.

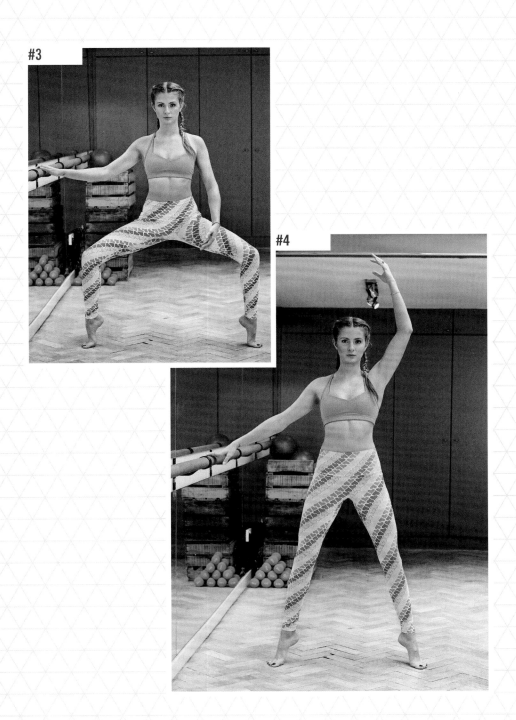

#3

#4

PBB DONKEY KICKS AT THE BARRE

This exercise works your lower back muscles, core, gluteal muscles and hamstrings.

#1

Facing the barre/chair back, rest your forearms along it with your hands overlapping each other. Drop your shoulders down and back and rise to demi pointe (onto the balls of your feet), making sure that you keep your waist pulled up and your stomach pulled in.

#2

Lift your right knee in towards your chest and then push your leg back, lifting it up behind you with your knee bent at a 90-degree angle and your thigh parallel with the floor. Squeeze your glutes as you lift, making sure you keep a neutral spine (not twisted to either side) and your hips square.

#3

Repeat 20 times, ending with 15 upward pulses with your foot flexed.

#4

Repeat on the other side.

#5

As an optional extra, load each leg with a 1–2kg weight or ball, squeezed behind the knee joint.

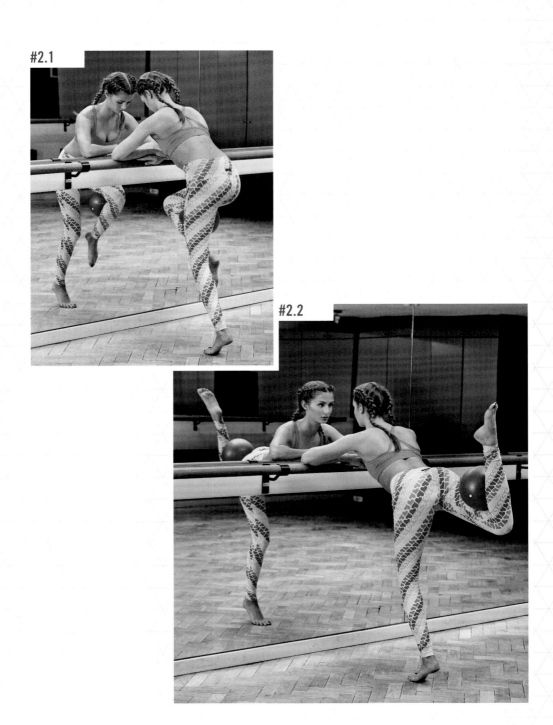

#2.1

#2.2

PBB ATTITUDE LIFTS DEVANT

This exercise works on the inner thighs and hips.

#1

Standing side on to the barre/chair back and with your right hand resting softly on it, place your feet in first position (heels together and feet turned out) and raise your heels off the floor to demi pointe (the balls of your feet).

#2

Raise your left arm in fifth position (above your head and with your hand curving in).

#3

Keeping your right leg long and lengthened and pulling your knees up to stabilise you, slide your left foot forward, toes pointed, and lift into 'attitude' position. Your lifted leg should be well turned out and bent at around 90 degrees. Your free arm should be lowered to second position (stretched out level with your shoulder and hand).

#4

Tap the toes of your left foot back down to the starting position, then repeat the exercise 15–20 times, ending with 15–20 upward pulses. Make sure you keep the knee of your lifted leg turned out at all times.

#5

Repeat on the other side.

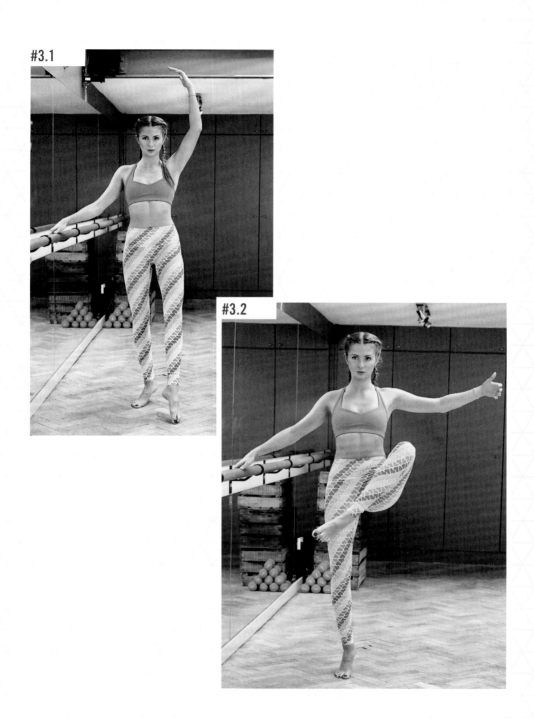

#3.1

#3.2

PBB STANDING SPLIT STRETCH OR ARABESQUE

This exercise will strengthen your glutes and back muscles and lengthen the hamstrings.

#1

Stand facing the barre/chair back with your arms fully extended and your hands (placed more than a shoulder width apart) holding it.

#2

Walk both feet back until you are bent over with your legs straight and your feet positioned directly under your hips. Make sure to keep your back flat and your chest pushed down towards the floor.

#3

Slide your right foot back, then lift your leg as high as it will go, squeezing your glutes as you lift.

#4

Slowly lower your leg back down, tapping your toes on the floor, and then dynamically lift the leg, so that you can feel the stretch in the back of your left leg. Make sure your hips don't twist as you kick but remain squarely aligned at all times.

#5

Repeat 15–20 times, ending with 15–20 upward pulses.

#6

Repeat on the other side.

#7

As an optional extra, this exercise can be done letting go of the barre/chair and lifting the chest up so the back goes into extension, improving balance and increasing back strength.

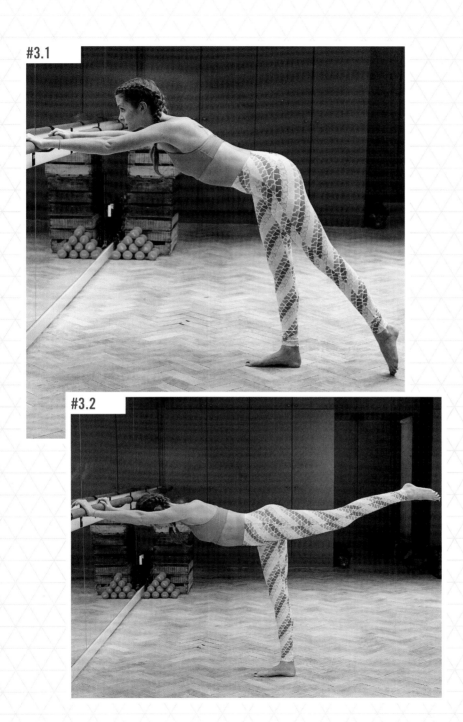

#3.1

#3.2

PBB KICK-BOXING BALLERINA

One of Paola's signature exercises, this works the glutes, waist and hips.

#1
Standing side on to the barre/chair back, rest your right forearm along it and place your left hand over your right. Rotate you right foot outwards by 45 degrees, then raise your left leg as high as you can so that it's parallel, or almost parallel, with the floor. Your hip, knee and toes should all be in alignment.

#2
Draw your left knee in towards your armpit, then press your leg out to full extension. (To keep control of the movement, imagine you're pushing through treacle.)

#3
Repeat ten times with flexed toes, then point your toes and do ten more. End with 10–20 lateral upward pulses in full extension position.

#4
Repeat on the other side.

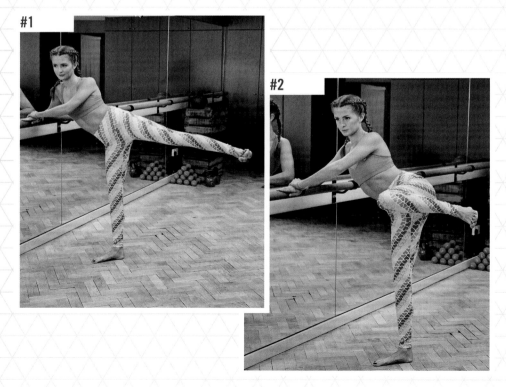

BOOT CAMP

Boot camps force you to challenge yourself with a range of different exercises that improve your overall fitness. There are loads available during the spring, summer and autumn and they are often set in beautiful countryside, but don't be fooled – boot camps are not retreats! Most last for a week and consist of a daily programme of agility courses, circuit-training sessions, hikes, relays and runs. You will be up early and dropping off over your super-healthy supper. But you will come back fitter, leaner and full of motivation to continue practising what you've learned.

BOXING

I never thought that boxing would suit me because of my bad co-ordination and lanky arms, but I love it. It gives a great cardio blast that burns fat from all over your body. Obviously, it's great for building strength in your arms and shoulders, but it's good for your core and legs too. I also find that it's a serious brain workout – you have to remember different combinations of punches and you're constantly defending and ducking.

I work with a trainer, but there are lots of classes around the country, such as those offered by Boxfit. I do think you should do a class initially because you need to learn the basic boxing stance, along with a few punches and how to throw them, but if you take a friend you can start doing it together at home once you've got the hang of it. One tip – long nails and boxing are not compatible: you can feel them bend inside the gloves as if they might snap at any minute.

PILATES

Dating back to the early 1900s, Pilates has stuck around for a reason: it works. It might remind you of your mum's corny workout videos, but the fantastic-looking Jane Fonda knew what she was talking about: Pilates provides a brilliant full-body type of exercise and is particularly good for the core and that stubborn mid-section. It also improves balance, muscle strength, flexibility and posture. There are two basic types:

 # MAT PILATES – which is good for core strength and ideal for beginners. One of the things I love about mat Pilates is that it really slows the exercises down and allows you to focus on getting the correct posture so that you activate the right muscles. All you need is an exercise mat, and if you can't get to a class, there are plenty on-line tutorials you can follow. I've included four exercises to get you started (see pages 251–254), which should all be done with Pilates breathing (see page 237).

 # PILATES REFORMER – a reformer is a flat bed with weighted springs, cables and straps that allows you to do the exercises from a variety of different positions. The added resistance can provide a tougher strength and endurance workout than a mat session. I'd advise you to use a reformer in a class or under supervision at the gym until you are confident that you know what you're doing.

FOREARM PLANK

The plank works your abs and back muscles. Adding the leg lift will increase the load on the core and work the glutes too.

#1

Start in a push-up position on the mat. Lower both your forearms to the ground so that your elbows are directly under your shoulders. Your palms can face up or down, but if you feel any tension in the space between your neck and shoulders, then you may find keeping your palms facing up is more comfortable. Draw your shoulders down and back, sending your shoulder blades into your 'back pockets'. Keep your neck lengthened with the crown of your head reaching forward.

#2

Squeeze your glutes and keep your hips in neutral (neither arched nor rounded). With every out breath, draw your navel towards your spine and keep as rigid as you can. (Imagine your body is a plank of wood or an arrow.) Hold this position for 30–60 seconds.

#3

As an optional extra, you can add a leg lift, lengthening and lifting one leg at a time. Repeat the leg lifts, alternating each leg, 10–20 times.

#2

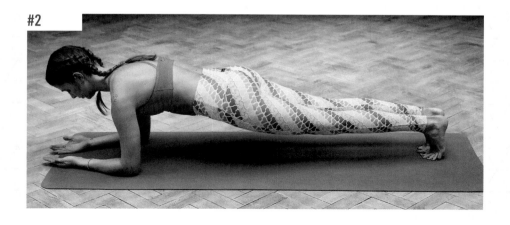

LOWER ABDOMINAL CRUNCHES

This exercise targets deep into the lower abdominal and rectus abdominis (six-pack) muscles, along with the shoulders and upper back.

#1

Sit up right on your bottom on the mat with your feet in alignment and your hips and legs bent, then draw your navel to your backbone and lower yourself to your elbows (which should be positioned directly under your shoulders) by rolling segmentally through the spine. Keep your chest open without arching your back.

#2

On an in-breath through the nose, raise one leg up, keeping it bent at a 90-degree angle at the knee. Exhale through the mouth and repeat so both legs are raised and bent at 90 degrees (start position).

#3

Extend both legs to 45 degrees, inhaling and squeezing the inner thighs as you go, then exhale as you draw both legs back into the start position.

#4

Repeat 15–20 times.

#5

To increase the load and difficulty, try coming off your elbows and onto just your hands. Keep your fingers facing forwards and your elbows bent halfway.

#3

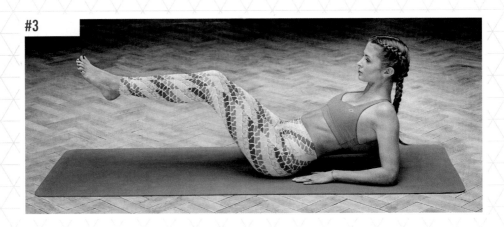

SIDE PLANK WITH LATERAL LEG LIFT

This exercise works both the core and oblique (side) muscles, improving overall strength and stability.

#1

Place your left hand on the mat, directly under your shoulder, then extend both legs out so that your body is in one straight line and you are balancing on the outside edge of your left foot. Rest your top hand on your hip or extend it into the air.

#2

Keeping your backbone long and lengthened, draw your navel towards your spine on a deep in-breath and lift your upper leg just higher than your top hip. Inhale as you slowly lower it back down to the bottom leg.

#3

Repeat 10–15 times on each side.

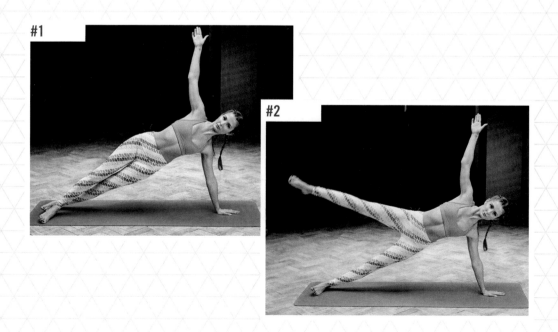

#1

#2

CRISS-CROSS CRUNCHES

This is a great core-strengthening exercise, targeting both your rectus abdominis and oblique muscles.

#1

Lie on your back with your knees bent at 90 degrees, your hands interlaced behind your head and your elbows wide. Keep your legs bent at the knees as you lift your shoulders off the floor with a deep inhalation. (Try not to pull on your head – you want to work the abdominal muscles, not the ones in your neck.)

#2

Exhale, pulling your navel towards your spine, and draw your right shoulder towards your left knee, holding your other leg straight.

#3

Slowly lower yourself again until your shoulders touch the ground and then repeat with the opposite side of your body, drawing your left shoulder towards you right knee.

#4

Repeat 20–30 times.

#2

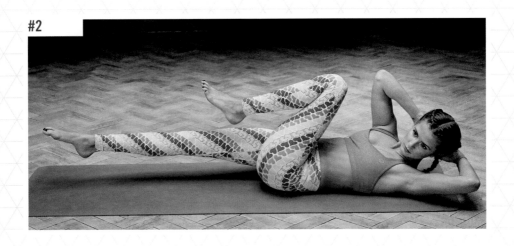

SKINNY BITCH COLLECTIVE (SBC)

This is an awesome class in London run by my friend Russell Bateman. It's become the go-to class for supermodels and is probably one of the most talked-about wellness and lifestyle regimes for women right now. But it's not just a fad; it really works. Russ has coached athletes and trained alongside some of Britain's top health professionals and his Skinny Bitch Collective is all about promoting a lean, strong body to help empower you as a woman. The 50-minute class is designed to throw you as far away from your comfort zone as possible – Russ's signature movements include upside-down burpees and lots of crawling on all fours – but the concept stretches into every aspect of your life (see page 270 for a list of the basic rules). SBC is about a balanced lifestyle and embraces elements that Russ believes will upgrade every aspect of your life. You can sum up his philosophy as squatting, sleep and sex! I love it; it really helps me to train the RIGHT way and, combined with my eating regime (see 'Food', pages 146–227), helps me feel great both inside and out.

SBC classes are invitation only, but here are eleven typical SBC/Millie exercises that you can do in the comfort of your home, using nothing but your own body. Work through the exercises in turn, resting for 29 seconds between each one. Aim to repeat the full circuit five times.

SBC CRAWL STAR JUMP

This is a great routine to engage all your muscle groups in preparation for a full workout. It also opens up the hips to allow for greater stability as you exercise.

#1

Squat down as low as you can, making sure that your chest is out and your shoulders are pulled back. Then walk your hands out in front of you until your body is stretched out fully while supported on your hands and bent toes, as if you were about to do a push-up.

#2

Walk your hands back to your start position and then transition into a star jump, twisting as you land so that you're facing the opposite direction. Keep your knees soft when you land (think of a cat), but try to be as explosive as possible when you jump.

#3

Immediately proceed to next crawl out in the opposite direction and proceed back to the start point for your jump and twist.

#4

Repeat 12–15 times, facing a different direction each time.

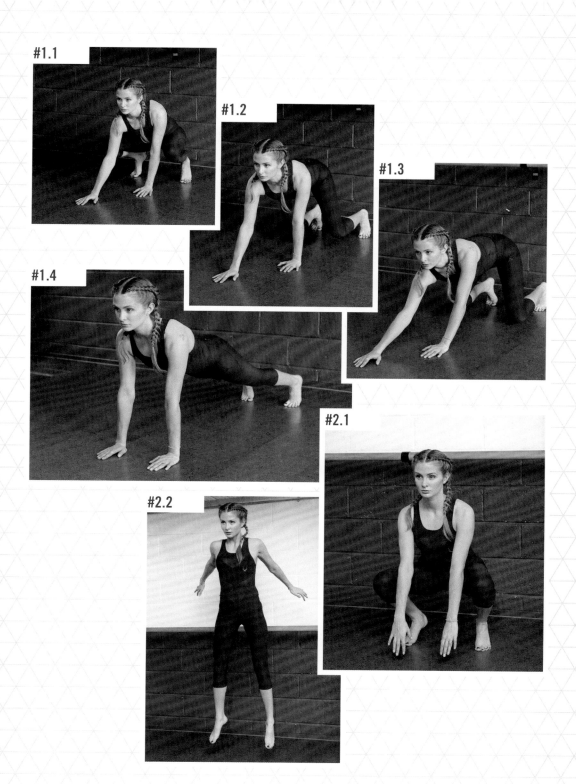

#1.1

#1.2

#1.3

#1.4

#2.1

#2.2

SBC CLOCK LUNGES

This is another good preparation exercise. The SBC clock lunges are designed to take your legs and your brain in different directions and to fire up the glutes, core and thighs.

#1

Imagine that you are in the centre of a clock. With your hands in the air, dynamically lunge forwards on your right leg to 12 o'clock, then backwards on the same leg to 6, sideways to 3 and to the opposite side for 9 (this final position looking like a curtsey).

#2

Repeat on the other side, repeating the exercise ten times, alternating from one leg to the other.

The knowledge that my body is strong enables me to believe in myself a bit more

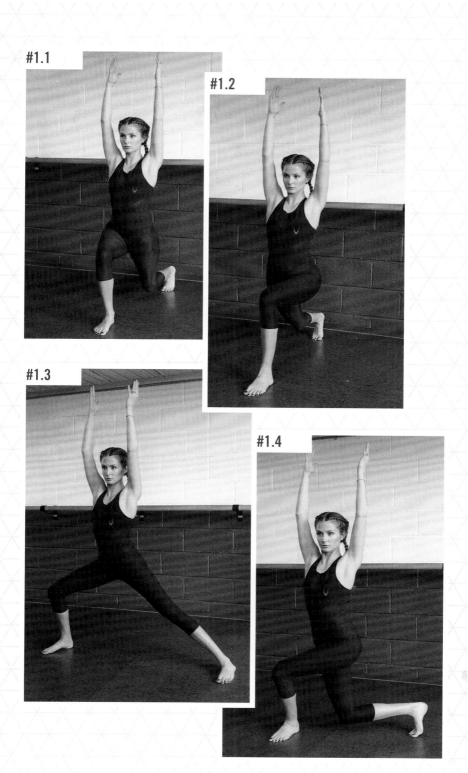

#1.1

#1.2

#1.3

#1.4

SBC BAND AID

This exercise, which uses a leg resistance band, activates the glutes and is good for really firing up the muscles before you go into a more intense routine.

#1

Attach the band directly below your knees. With your left hand resting on a barre/chair back and your right arm outstretched to the side, rise up onto your toes.

#2

Keeping as much tension as possible, pull your right leg as far away from your left leg as you can.

#3

Hold for 5 seconds.

#4

Repeat 12–15 times on each side.

#1

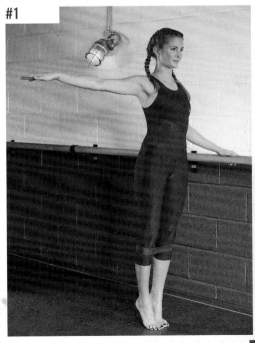

#2

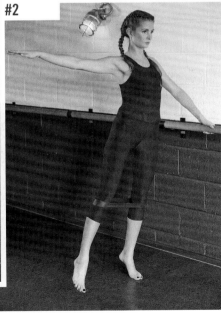

SBC WALL CLIMBERS

This is a good cardio exercise that works your shoulders and core. Brain function and co-ordination are key here as well.

#1

Begin in a semi handstand against a wall. Keeping your body aligned and your core tight, pull your left knee into your tummy. Immediately stretch your leg out again and pull in your right knee.

#2

Keep pumping with alternating knees, making sure that your body is straight and your glutes and core are engaged at all times. You should also try and squeeze you shoulder blades together as you pump your legs – and don't forget to breathe!

#3

Repeat for 15–20 seconds.

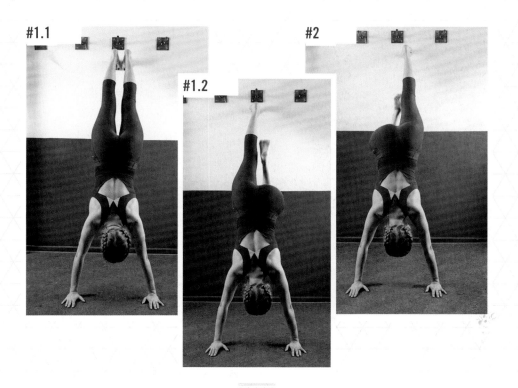

#1.1

#1.2

#2

SBC CANCAN KICKS

A great cardio workout, this exercise works your core, glutes and triceps.

#1
Get yourself into a crab-walk position, then push your palms down, keeping your hips strong and quite high but also allowing for some 'bounce'.

#2
Alternating from one leg to the other, explosively kick each foot as high as you can, while squeezing your triceps as tightly as possible.

#3
Repeat for 30 seconds.

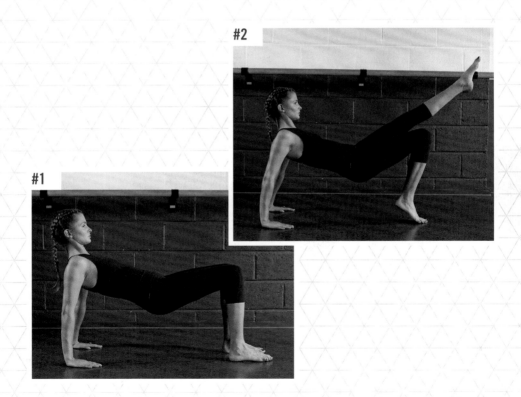

#2

#1

SBC SINGLE-LEG GLUTE RAISE

This exercise works the glutes, the hamstrings and the posterior chain muscles.

#1

Lie on the floor with your knees bent and feet flat. Raise one leg off the ground, pulling it towards to your chest. This is your starting position.

#2

Push your bent leg forwards by driving through the heel, extending your hip upwards and raising your glutes off the ground. Extend as far as possible, pause and then return to the starting position.

#3

Repeat 30 times, alternating from one leg to the other.

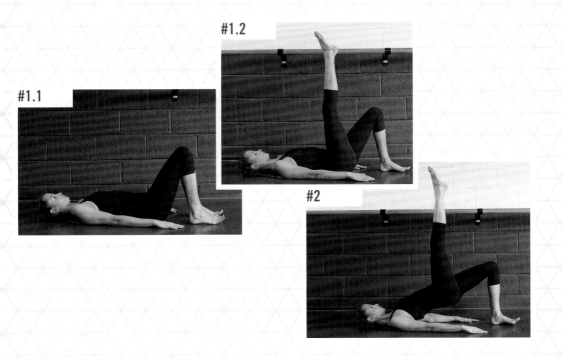

#1.2

#1.1

#2

SBC DEEP SQUAT

This exercise works the glutes, thighs, calves, abs and heart.

#1

Standing with your feet apart and on tiptoe, take a deep breath, contract your abs and descend. It should feel like you are sitting back on a chair behind you; not going straight down. Keep your knees in line with your feet and raise your arms out in front of you for balance. You should start your descent at the knees, not the hips. Control your descent and maintain tightness in the upper back through the movement.

#2

Try to go as low as you can without your back collapsing in on itself and then drive yourself up, pushing through your heels.

#3

Repeat 15 times.

#1.1

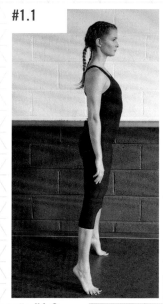

#1.2

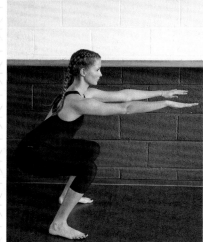

SBC LEG RAISES

This exercise works your abdominals and lower back.

#1

Place your hands under your glutes with your palms facing down and your legs raised a few inches above the floor. Keeping your legs as straight as possible (hold a dumbbell between your feet if you want added resistance), slowly raise them until they are perpendicular to the floor. Hold the contraction at the top for a second, then slowly lower your legs to the start position.

#2

Repeat 15 times, never letting your feet touch the floor between raises.

#3

As an optional extra, raise one leg at a time, holding the contraction at the top as in step 1 and alternating from one leg to the other 30 times.

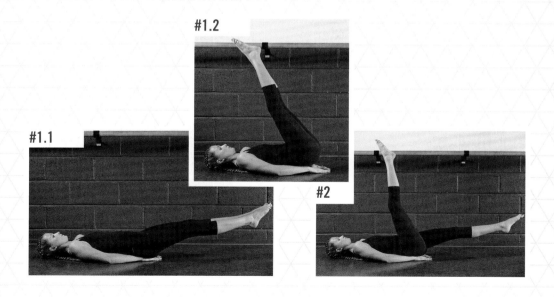

#1.2

#1.1

#2

SBC PUSH-UP RAISES

This exercise works the chest, triceps and core and helps to improve your balance.

#1

Lie face down on the floor, ready to get into push-up position. Push yourself up from the floor, engaging your core and glutes – your back should be straight and your arms locked out.

#2

From this position, lift your left arm and right leg together and hold for 2 seconds.

#3

Lower your left arm and right leg to the floor and repeat with the opposite arm and leg, holding for 2 seconds.

#4

Repeat the whole exercise 12–15 times.

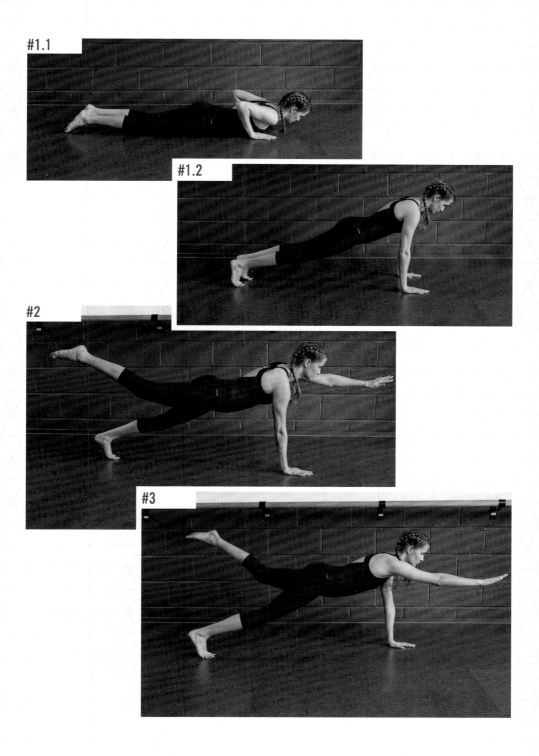

SBC SQUAT KICK-OUTS

This one is great for the butt, legs and abs and gives a good cardio workout too.

#1

Holding a barre or the back of a chair with both hands, take a deep breath, contract your abs and descend, keeping your knees in line with your feet and starting the descent at the knees not the hips. (As with the Deep Squat on page 264, it should feel as if you're sitting back on a chair behind you, rather than going straight down.) Control your descent and maintain tightness in the upper back through the movement.

#2

Try to go as low as you can without your back collapsing in on itself, and then drive up, pushing through your heels. Rise up explosively, kicking your legs out to the side as far as they will go when you jump.

#3

Repeat 12–15 times.

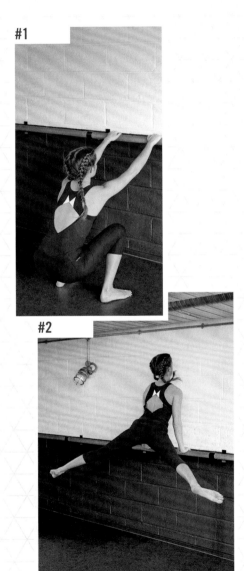

\#1

\#2

SBC SINGLE LEG ROW

This exercise works the biceps, back and the stabiliser muscles in your legs to really improve your balance. If you don't have any dumb-bells, try a couple of full water bottles.

#1

Standing with your feet a shoulder width apart and holding a dumb-bell/bottle in each hand, bend over until your torso is almost parallel with the floor.

#2

Allow the dumb-bells/bottles to hang at arm's length from your shoulders with your palms facing each other. Keeping your lower back naturally arched, slightly bend your knees and raise your right leg behind you.

#3

Hold for 2 seconds, then pull your arms into your sides in a rowing motion, making sure you squeeze in your shoulder blades and raise and lower your arms at a slow and controlled tempo.

#4

Repeat 12–15 times.

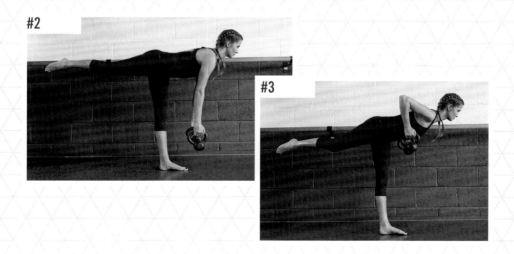

#2

#3

SBC RULES FOR LIFE

SWEAT AND MOVE DAILY – it doesn't matter what you do – dance, walk, sex, yoga, Pilates, SBC workout – just do it!

EAT RAW AS MUCH AS POSSIBLE – raw, organic, vegan food is best for our DNA. Buy a cold-press juicer – it will change your life!

STAY IN THE NOW AS MUCH AS YOU CAN.

MAKE SURE YOUR BREATHING IS FULL AND DEEP – it's the best detox.

LOVE YOURSELF UNCONDITIONALLY – or you can never love anyone else unconditionally.

MIX UP YOUR WORKOUTS – for the good of your body and your brain.

BE AS CHILDLIKE AS POSSIBLE – embrace your inner five-year-old.

DON'T JUDGE – judgement is just so boring!

TAKE NOTHING – even the stuff directed towards you – personally.

EARLY TO BED – on nights in, go to bed by 10 p.m.

BE IN NATURE AS MUCH AS POSSIBLE.

THROW AWAY YOUR TV AND READ MORE.

DANCING IS NOT A LUXURY – it's an imperative. Start your day with a morning dance.

COCONUT BUTTER! – eat it and moisturise and clean your teeth with it.

ANYTHING CAN BE A MEDITATION – (walking, yoga, cooking, sex, taking out the rubbish) just be present.

STRIVE TO RAISE YOUR VIBRATION DAILY.

SMILE!

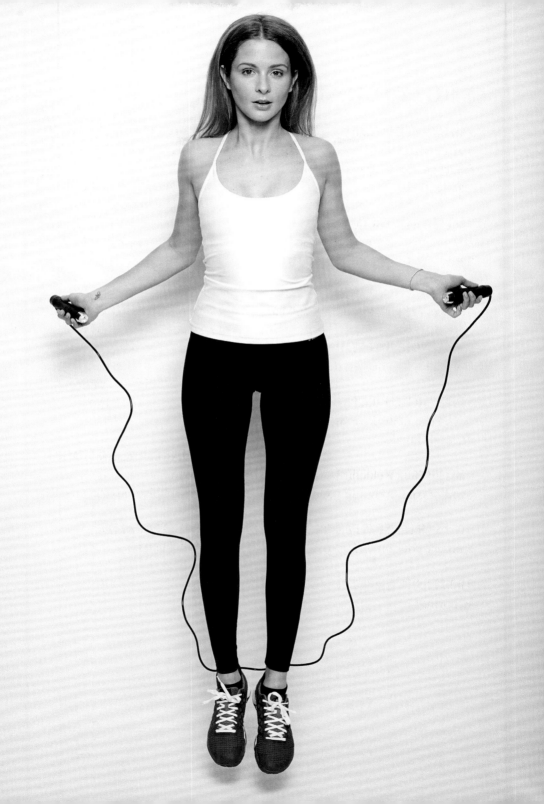

SPINNING

Spinning (cycling at high speed on a static bike) is a great cardio workout and is especially good for toning your legs and bum. With the right music, it's a good stress buster too.

Some women think that spinning bulks up your legs and it does depend a bit on your body type, but if you're doing it right, the pressure should be taken out of your thighs because you have to cycle with your heel and push and pull with your feet. Of course, cycling through the park with the wind in your hair is lovely, but in a class the sprints and hill climbs are specifically designed to ensure that you burn fat as effectively as possible. And you're given light weights so your shoulders get a workout too.

I got into SoulCycle while I was in America. You do it in a very dark room with disco lights and rise up and down from your seat in time to the beat. It's great fun and the trainer doubles as a DJ. In this country, I go to Psycle and Flywheel, which are similar. Spinning is quite intense, so classes tend to last for only 45 minutes – ideal if you're in a hurry.

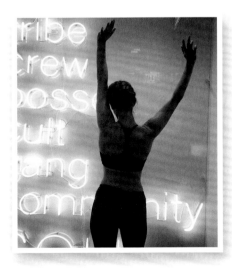

WEIGHTS

Weights don't make you manly, girls! I resisted the idea of weights at first because I didn't want to get too muscly, but I've discovered that all they do is to improve tone.

My weight sessions – which are basically exercise classes with the added pressure of lifting weights – target either my upper or my lower body. (You can do full body sessions using lighter weights but I find that targeted ones work better for me.) In a week I would ideally do one targeting each part of my body. Legs days are my absolute worst – they really make my muscles burn. (Regular exercise puts you in touch with your body, so you start to tell the difference between the kind of muscle soreness that comes from a good workout and the achiness caused by overdoing it. If you suspect the latter, then you need to ease off.) I would recommend going to a weights class initially because you need to get the correct posture and grip so that you don't hurt yourself. If you can't find a class, you can go the gym and ask one of their trainers to show you the right positions.

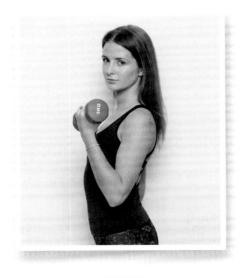

YOGA

I wish I had paid attention in those sixth-form classes because I now enjoy yoga and would love to be better at it. Some of the exercises I do can shorten my muscles and a weekly yoga class helps to stretch them out again and keep me flexible. There are lots of different types, but these are the ones I enjoy:

HOT YOGA

Hot yoga is yoga in a studio heated to around 38°C (just above body temperature). The heat helps your muscles, ligaments and tendons to stretch, and because it makes you sweat, it's cleansing too. There's something incredibly restorative about hot yoga when it's cold outside and I also like to do it when I feel in need of a detox. I either do a basics class, in which the teacher explains the benefits of each pose as you do it, or a flow class – where, rather than stopping between poses, you flow slowly from one to the next.

JIVAMUKTI

One of the nine internationally recognised styles of hatha yoga, Jivamukti taps in to the spiritual aspects of yoga as much as the physical practice. I stumbled across it by mistake and hadn't realised that it involved a lot of chanting, but to my surprise, I loved it.

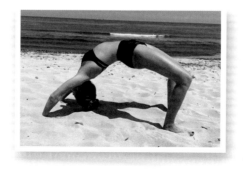

I found letting go of my inhibitions quite a spiritual, cleansing experience. The classes are mixed ability and you just do each pose the best you can.

YIN YOGA

This is designed to target the connective tissues in the pelvis, hips and lower spine, areas that aren't worked in other styles of yoga. It's very slow – in the class I go to, we hold each pose for about three minutes, but it can be as long as 20 minutes in some classes. Resistance work and weight training can shorten muscles, so I try to do a yin yoga class once a week to stretch myself out again. I also find it a good way to recover from the stresses of the week.

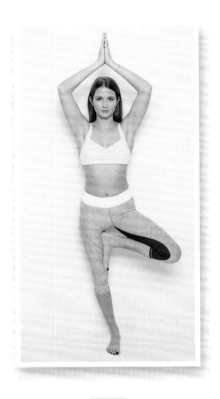

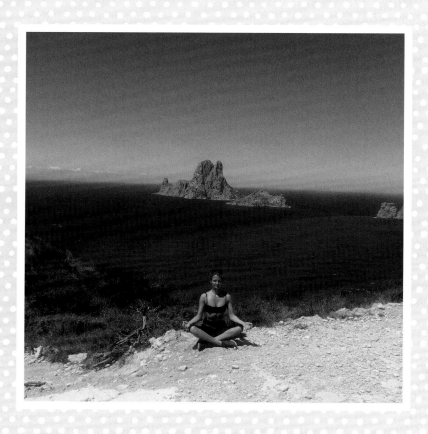

STRESS RELIEF

Stress is a natural reaction to something we find threatening or challenging, but while a small amount is beneficial, keeping us on our toes, too much stress is incredibly bad for us. It makes us tired, accelerates ageing (especially in women – how unfair is that?), impairs the immune system, raises blood pressure and can even cause fat cells to accumulate around the abdomen, leading to an increased risk of having a heart attack or stroke. Stress is hard to avoid, so the only solution is to learn how to manage it better.

I have suffered from stress-related anxiety attacks for several years and they can be disabling. My stomach goes to jelly and I feel that I can't breathe. However, I have found several ways to prevent attacks coming on in the first place and to reduce them on those occasions when they still strike.

BREATHING

Focusing on your breathing will help you to calm your mind. These are two breathing exercises I do if I feel my stress and anxiety levels building when I'm out and about.

#1

Inhale deeply. (Put your hands on your tummy so you can feel the breath being drawn deep into your stomach.) Hold for a few seconds then exhale, making sure you breathe all the air out. Take it slowly and repeat ten times.

#2

Count your breaths up to ten – an inhale and an exhale counts as one – and repeat.

MEDITATION

I got into meditation through the mind–body specialist Graham Doke. I had been seeing a doctor about my anxiety but it wasn't really getting me anywhere, so I thought I would try meditation. My first guided session with Graham was incredible: I just listened to his voice and concentrated on my breathing as he got me to visualise myself climbing a mountain, and I really did reach this place of pure bliss, calm and emptiness. I find meditation clears my mind, enabling me to take on more and cope better with stressful situations.

I do still go and see Graham when I can, but I also use his free app, Anamaya, which has 350 different meditations covering eleven different areas to focus on, from stress and anxiety to pain and anger. This is my home meditation routine. As with any workout, practice makes perfect. The more you do, the longer you'll be able to keep going: start at 10 minutes and build from there.

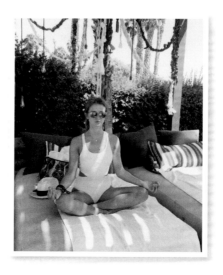

SIMPLE, DAILY MEDITATION

#1
Find a quiet, comfortable place and make this your special meditation spot.

#2
Sit with your spine straight, your legs crossed and your hands resting on your knees. This posture stops you falling asleep and helps to keep your mind focused.

#3
Close your eyes.

#4
Close your mouth, relax your jaw and breathe through your nostrils.

#5
Inhale and exhale slowly three or four times, focusing on the sensation of breathing.

#6
I switch on the app at this point, but you can simply sit, focusing on your breathing.

#7
If you feel your mind wandering, just return to step 5 and focus on your breathing.

#8
If you are using the app, it will bring you out of the meditation at this point. If not, just sit for a moment and assess how you are feeling and the emotions you have experienced during the meditation.

ACUPUNCTURE

Once a month, I have a facial with acupuncture, which involves having needles inserted into my eyebrows, scalp and ears. It doesn't hurt but you can feel the pressure and I find that it releases all the tension in my face. Nataliya Robinson also places magnets on my ears when she is giving me a facial, as the ears have pressure points. I pinch these pressure points when I feel stressed to try to calm myself.

REIKI

I gave Reiki a go the day before my first appearance at the BAFTAs. I was super-stressed and found it did help. The therapist, Elizabeth Caroline, moved her hands over me and I could feel the heat and energy coming off them without her even touching me. It released a lot of emotion and I left feeling much calmer. The healer will read your energy and chakrus. It helps to slow everything down.

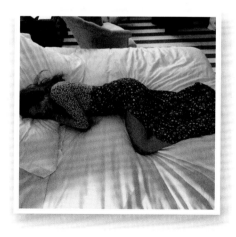

REST

Your body needs time to repair itself, so it's important to build some rest days into your routine. I aim to work out five times a week, but I would never do more than three days in succession. I learned the hard way, pushing myself to train every day and eventually turning up to sessions so tired I may as well not have bothered. A rest day means just that – don't think of doing anything other than some gentle stretching. I also like to take a whole week off a couple of times a year.

Don't underestimate the power of a good night's sleep. Being tired not only leaves you lethargic and grumpy, it also makes you crave high-calorie foods. I need a good seven hours a night and I'm usually so tired that I have no problem falling asleep. But like everyone, there are times when I can't drop off, so here are my tips for getting to sleep:

★ Go to bed early and read – or better still, get someone to read to you. Take a book rather than an e-reader or a laptop as the light from the screen sends messages to your body that it's daytime.

★ Soak in a bath of magnesium flakes. It not only makes you relax, but the minerals help to rid your muscles of the lactic acid that builds up during exercise.

★ Lie on your back with your hands on your stomach and breathe deeply, drawing your breath right down into your tummy. Breathe out, pushing every last drop of air from your body. Repeat ten times.

★ Follow a bedtime routine so your body knows that it's time to sleep.

★ Try a meditation tape that targets sleep.

DIRECTORIES

STYLE

HIGH-STREET:

Gap www.gap.co.uk – Great for staple t-shirts.

H & M www.hm.com/gb

Mango shop.mango.com/GB – This is a nice
shop for one-offs and statement pieces.

Marks & Spencer www.marksandspencer.com

Miss Selfridge www.missselfridge.com
– Stocks stunning party pieces.

River Island www.riverisland.com
– Great for jeans and strappy sandals.

Topshop www.topshop.com

Zara www.zara.com/uk
– Perfect for basics, shoes and jewellery.

HIGHER END:

Anthropologie www.anthropologie.com
– Great for jewellery and homewear.

A.P.C. www.apc.fr/wwuk/women_u1.html

Baar & Bass baarandbass.com – For cool t-shirts,
jeans, beach clothing and amazing jewellery.

By Malene Birger www.bymalenebirger.com/gb

Citizens of Humanity
www.citizensofhumanity.com

Donna Ida www.donnaida.com
– A denim boutique and great for blouses too.

Drome www.drome.co.uk
– Amazing leather trousers.

Farfetch www.farfetch.com

James Perse www.jamesperse.com
– Fabulous t-shirts.

J Brand www.jbrandjeans.com

J.Crew www.jcrew.com

Madewell www.madewell.com

Maje uk.maje.com
– Statement pieces and easy to wear items.

MOTHER www.motherdenim.com

Mother of Pearl www.motherofpearl.co.uk

Paige Jeans www.paige.com

Rails www.railsclothing.com – Super plaid shirts.

Sandro uk.sandro-paris.com – Shop here for a
statement coat or an easy to wear dress or suit.

Sass & Bide www.sassandbide.com

Sundry sundryclothing.com
– Stocks great sweats.

The Kooples www.thekooples.co.uk
– Wonderful suits and blazers.

The Shop at Bluebird
www.theshopatbluebird.com

Theory www.theory.com

Zuhair Murad www.zuhairmurad.com

202 www.202london.com

DESIGNER (JUST A FEW OF MY FAVOURITES!):

Acne Studios www.acnestudios.com
– Amazing leather jackets and simple pieces,
good for dresses, shoes and jeans too.

Alexander Wang www.alexanderwang.com

Burberry uk.burberry.com – For coats and shoes.

Chanel www.chanel.com/en_GB – A classic
choice for handbags, sunglasses and shoes.

Helmut Lang www.helmutlang.com
– Easy to wear, well cut pieces.

Isabel Marant www.isabelmarant.com/en
– The clothes my dreams are made of!

Joseph www.joseph-fashion.com
– Great for coats and worth waiting for a sale!

Matthew Williamson www.matthewwilliamson.
com – For prints and stand out pieces.

Stella McCartney www.stellamccartney.com/gb
– Mini dresses, sports wear, underwear…
actually, all of it!

Valentino www.valentino.com/gb
– The most fabulous shoes and dream dresses
that I can only admire from afar.

Victoria Beckham www.victoriabeckham.com
– Fabulous dresses.

DEPARTMENT STORES:

Harrods www.harrods.com

Harvey Nichols www.harveynichols.com

Liberty www.liberty.co.uk

Selfridges www.selfridges.com

ONLINE:

ASOS www.asos.com
Girl Meets Dress www.girlmeetsdress.com
Grace Loves Lace www.etsy.com/uk/shop/
  Graceloveslace – For all things wedding.
Matches Fashion www.matchesfashion.com
Millie Mackintosh www.millie-mackintosh.com
Nasty Gal www.nastygal.com
Net-a-porter www.net-a-porter.com
Reformation www.thereformation.com
Shopbop www.shopbop.com
Stone Cold Fox thestonecoldfox.com

FOOTWEAR:

Alaia www.net-a-porter.com/Shop/Designers/
  Alaia
Ancient Greek Sandals www.ancient-greek-
  sandals.com
Ash Footwear www.ashfootwear.co.uk
  – Amazing ankle boots.
Charlotte Olympia www.charlotteolympia.com
Christian Louboutin www.christianlouboutin.
  com
Isabel Marant www.isabelmarant.com/en
Jimmy Choo row.jimmychoo.com/en/home
Kurt Geiger www.kurtgeiger.com
Office www.office.co.uk
River Island www.riverisland.com
Sam Edelman www.samedelman.com
  – Statement boots and shoes.
Stuart Weitzman www.stuartweitzman.com –
  Stunning shoes.
Stuart Weitzman for Russell & Bromley www.
  russellandbromley.co.uk
  – For heels and over the knee boots.
Valentino www.valentino.com/gb
Zara www.zara.com/uk

VINTAGE:

Beyond Retro www.beyondretro.com
Elvira Vintage www.elviravintage.com
One Vintage www.onevintagedesigns.com
Vintage to Vogue www.vintagetovoguebath.co.uk
  – Great antique clothes shop in Bath.
William Vintage www.williamvintage.com
  – Showroom and online.

SUNGLASSES:

ASOS www.asos.com – Fabulous
  budget sunnies.
Chanel www.chanel.com/en_GB
Dior www.dior.com/home/en_gb
Karen Walker www.karenwalker.com
Ray-Ban www.ray-ban.com/uk
The Row www.therow.com – Great selection.
Thierry Lasry www.thierrylasry.com

WORKOUT WEAR:

Adidas www.adidas.co.uk
Lorna Jane www.lornajane.com.au
Lucas Hugh www.lucashugh.com
Lulu Lemon www.lululemon.co.uk
Nike www.nike.com
Reebok www.reebok.co.uk
Stella McCartney for Adidas www.adidas.co.uk/
  adidas_by_stella_mccartney
Sweaty Betty www.sweatybetty.com
Victoria's Secret www.victoriassecret.com

UNDERWEAR:

Agent Provocateur www.agentprovocateur.com
ASOS www.asos.com
Calvin Klein www.calvinklein.com
Cheekfrills www.cheekfrills.co.uk
Coco de Mer www.coco-de-mer.com
Cosabella www.cosabella.com
Eberjey www.eberjey.com
Fleur of England www.fleurofengland.com
Hanky Panky www.hankypanky.com
Huit www.huit.com
Spanx www.spanx.com
Victoria's Secret www.victoriassecret.com

SLEEPWEAR:

Cheekfrills www.cheekfrills.co.uk
Eberjey www.eberjey.com
Fleur of England www.fleurofengland.com
Olivia von Halle oliviavonhalle.com
Rosie Huntington-Whiteley for Autograph
  www.marksandspencer.com/s/lingerie/
  rosie-for-autograph
The White Company www.thewhitecompany.com

SWIMWEAR AND COVER-UPS:

American Apparel americanapparel.co.uk
ASOS www.asos.com
B LONDON www.blondonboutique.com
Biondi Couture www.biondicouture.com
Emamò www.emamo.com
Heidi Klein www.heidiklein.com
Kiini kiini.com
Lisa Marie Fernandez www.lisamariefernandez.com
Melissa Odabash www.odabash.com
MIKOH www.mikoh.com
Monday Swimwear mondayswimwear.com
Salt Resort Wear www.saltresortwear.com
Triangl international.triangl.com/collections/
swimwear
V i X Paula Hermanny www.vixpaulahermanny.com
Zimmermann www.zimmermannwear.com

BEAUTY

SPAS:

Cavendish Clinic & Medispa
www.cavendishclinic.co.uk/medispa –
Provides laser hair removal.
Chelsea Private Clinic chelseaprivateclinic.com
– For colonic hydrotherapy, teeth whitening
and food intolerance testing.
Corinthia Spa www.espalifeatcorinthia.com
–You can go and just rest in their sleep pods,
so lovely to go with the girls or alone if you
really need some me time.
Mandarin Oriental www.mandarinoriental.com/
london/luxury-spa/Sanctuary Spa
www.sanctuary.com/en-gb

FACIALS:

Debbie Thomas www.debbiethomas.co.uk
– A facialist who is great with problem skin.
Elizabeth Caroline www.elizabethcaroline.co.uk
– Reiki healer who does facials and massage.
Nataliya Robinson www.nataliyarobinson.co.uk
– Provides amazing facial acupuncture.
Nichola Joss www.nicholajoss.com (14 Upper St
Martins Lane) – For the best facial massage,
lymphatic drainage and a great tan.

SALONS:

Bliss Spa www.blissworld.co.uk
– Fabulous oxygen facials.
Blow Ltd www.blowltd.com – Blow dry bar
which does make-up and nails all in an hour.
Cow Shed www.cowshedonline.com
– A great one-stop place for everything you
need. They do wonderful facials and massages.
Duck & Dry www.duckanddry.com
– A lovely blow dry bar.
Hershesons www.hershesons.com
– Hair, nails and a great braid bar.
Lockonego www.lockonego.com
– Great for hair cuts, colour and blow drys.
Rys Hair and Beauty www.ryshairandbeauty.com
– Stunning hair and nails.
Strip www.stripwaxbar.com – Good for waxing.

HAIR AND MAKE-UP ARTISTS:

Emily McEwan @Emily_McEwan
Jo Hamilton @jo_a_hamilton
Justine Jenkins @JJmakeup
Keash Braids www.keashbraids.co.uk
Louis Bryne @louisbyrnehair
Mark Hill www.markhill.co.uk
Miguel Martin Perez at Josh Wood Colour
@Miguapochino – Fabulous hair stylist.
Miguel did my wedding hair!
Scarlett Rainer @ScarlettRainer

AT HOME TREATMENTS:

Jules Heptonstall http://www.julesheptonstall.
com – Beauty consultant and tanning expert.
Lava Angels lavaangels.com – Hot stone
massage at home, amazingly relaxing.
Perfect 10 www.perfect10mobilebeauty.co.uk
– Perfect for pampering, they come to your
house to do all the beauty treatments.

MAKE-UP:

BECCA Cosmetics www.beccacosmetics.com
blinc www.blincinc.com
By Terry www.byterry.com
Chanel www.chanel.com/en_GB
Chantecaille Beauté www.chantecaille.com
Charlotte Tilbury www.charlottetilbury.com

Estee Lauder www.esteelauder.co.uk
Revlon www.revlon.co.uk
Smashbox www.smashbox.co.uk
Urban Decay www.urbandecay.co.uk
Yves Saint Laurent www.yslbeauty.co.uk

SKINCARE:

Feel Unique www.feelunique.com – online beauty.
Kiehl's www.kiehls.co.uk
Nurse Jamie nursejamie.com
Ren Skincare www.renskincare.com
Sarah Chapman www.sarahchapman.net
Sephora www.sephora.com
Space NK uk.spacenk.com – Beauty boutique.
Zelens Ltd www.zelens.com

FOOD

SHOPS:

Always go to your local farmers market on the
    weekend – you will find some wonderful items.
CPRESS www.cpressjuice.com
Marks & Spencer www.marksandspencer.com
Planet Organic www.planetorganic.com
Waitrose www.waitrose.com
Whole Foods Market www.wholefoodsmarket.com

ONLINE:

Abel & Cole: Organic Food Delivery
    www.abelandcole.co.uk
Chris James www.chrisjamesmindbody.com
Detox kitchen detoxkitchen.co.uk
Gousto www.gousto.co.uk
Graze: Healthy Snacks by Post www.graze.com/uk
HelloFresh www.hellofresh.co.uk
Hemsley + Hemsley
    www.hemsleyandhemsley.com – Fabulous
    healthy eating blog and cookbook.
Honestly Healthy honestlyhealthyfood.com
Purifyne Cleanse www.purifynecleanse.com
Riverford www.riverford.co.uk

RESTAURANTS/CAFES:

Hally's www.hallyslondon.com
    – Good for a fresh, healthy.

Jak's www.jakskingsroad.co.uk
    – Great for a take-away lunch that is full of
    protein and they do really yummy salads.
L'ETO Caffé letocaffe.co.uk
Nama Foods namafoods.com
    – Delicious raw food restaurant.
Natural Kitchen www.thenaturalkitchen.com
    – Also great for a clean take-away lunch.
Nobu www.noburestaurants.com
Ottolenghi www.ottolenghi.co.uk – Superb cafés.
R O K A www.rokarestaurant.com/www.
    rokarestaurant.com
    – Amazing Japanese restaurant.
Roots & Bulbs www.rootsandbulbs.com
The Chequers www.thechequersbath.com
    – Lovely pub in Bath, with a great Sunday lunch.
The Circus Café and Restaurant www.
    thecircuscafeandrestaurant.co.uk
    – Fabulous restaurant in Bath.
The Good Life Eatery www.goodlifeeatery.com
The Pig www.thepighotel.com/near-bath/explore
    – Hotel in Hunstrete that serves wonderful food.
202 www.202london.com
    – Café with an amazing boutique downstairs.

FITNESS

CLASSES:

Barrecore www.barrecore.co.uk
Boom Cycle www.boomcycle.co.uk
Flywheel www.flywheelsports.com
Frame www.moveyourframe.com
Graham Doke, Anamaya anamaya.co.uk
Lomax www.lomaxpt.com
Moreno Boxing www.morenoboxing.co.uk
Paola's BodyBarre www.paolasbodybarre.com
Psycle psyclelondon.com
Skinny Bitch Collective thesbcollective.com
The Model Method, PilatesPT www.pilatespt.co.uk
Triyoga www.triyoga.co.uk

APPS:

Class Pass classpass.com
Mindbody Connect www.mindbodyonline.com/connect

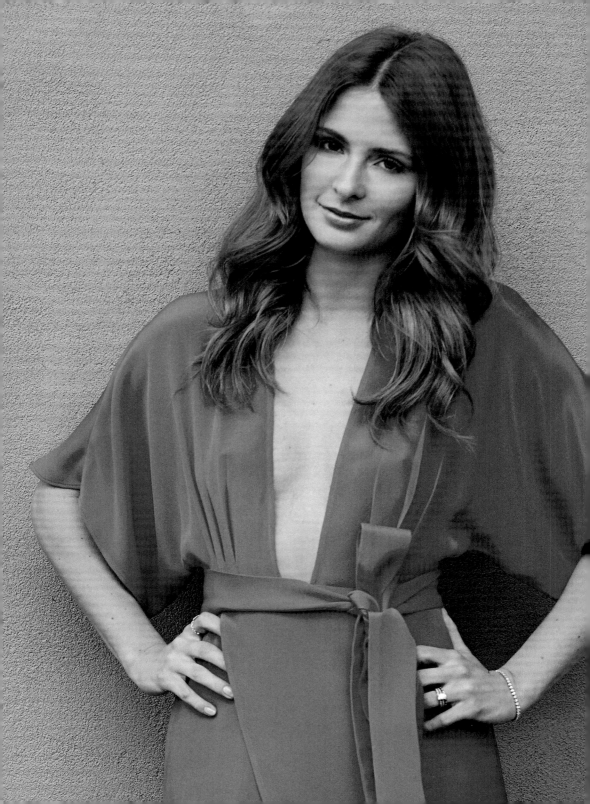

ACKNOWLEDGEMENTS

With many thanks to:

My mum, dad and sister for their love and support, always.

My grandparents for their wise words.

My best friends for always being there.

Stephen for making me a better person and keeping my feet on the ground.

My foodie friends Gizzi Erskine and Madeleine Shaw for all their advice and inspiration.

My agent Kirsty Reilly at Select Models, and my publicists Tim Beaumont and Emily Sherwood at Beaumont Communications.

Ebury for the chance to make this book!

Charlotte Abrahams, Dan Kennedy, Francesca Waddell, Frankie Unsworth, Kate Parker, Emma Lahaye and Smith & Gilmour.

Paola de Lanza at Paola's BodyBarre.

Russell Bateman at the Skinny Bitch Collective.

Mark Hill, Angie Smith, Natalya Robinson, Nichola Joss, Louis Byrne, Justine Jenkins, Jo Hamilton, Emily McEwan, Soho House and Taiba at Keash Braids.

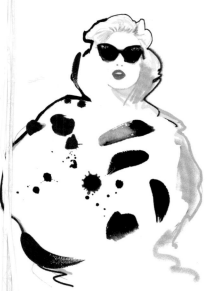

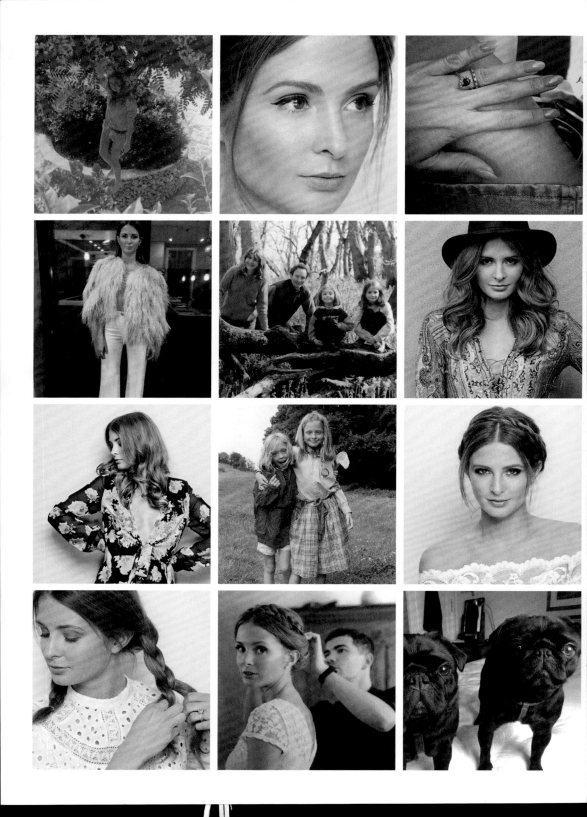